Designing a Health Care Corporate Compliance Program

David D. Queen
Elizabeth Ellen Frasher

*Attorneys With the Law Firm of
Ober, Kaler, Grimes & Shriver*

Edited By

David Mlawsky
Phoebe Eliopoulos

Atlantic Information Services, Inc.
1100 17th Street, NW, Suite 300 • Washington, D.C. 20036 • (202) 775-9008

This publication is designed to provide accurate, comprehensive and authoritative information on the subject matter covered. However, the publisher does not warrant that information contained herein is complete or accurate. This book is published with the understanding that the publisher is not engaged in rendering legal or other professional services. If legal advice or other expert assistance is required, the services of a competent professional person should be sought.

ISBN: 0-929156-09-9

For reprint permission, or information regarding individual or bulk purchases, contact: Atlantic Information Services, Inc., 1100 17th Street, NW, Suite 300, Washington, D.C. 20036 (1-800-521-4323; 202-775-9008).

Table of Contents

Preface

Our aim in writing this book is to offer a practical overview of the important topic of corporate compliance in the most heavily regulated industry in America. It is written as a practical guide for lawyers and non-lawyers alike who work in the health care field. Hence, footnotes and case citations have been kept to a minimum. At the end of each chapter, however, we have included a list of additional resources.

This book was written with the assumption that the reader has little familiarity with the subject of corporate compliance programs. Consequently, it explains what a compliance program is and why your organization needs one.

As the following chapters will demonstrate, a corporate compliance program is necessary, affordable, even indispensable to any health care organization. Whether yours is a small medical practice, a billing service, a laboratory or a large corporate health care provider, a compliance program is a must.

Many in-house counsel, auditors and others responsible for assuring that an organization does not violate the law find their first problem is convincing the board of directors and officers of the importance of a compliance program. Outside counsel often complain that their biggest problem is convincing the client and even in-house counsel of the need to adopt a program. The following chapters contain arguments useful in conveying to skeptical clients, employees and boards the need for a compliance program.

Consequently, this book is organized to address the "why" questions before addressing the "what" and "how" of corporate compliance.

Readers already familiar with the purpose of a corporate compliance program, and already sold on its benefits, will find practical information on how to design and implement an effective program.

Atlantic Information Services Inc. wishes to express its gratitude to the book's authors, David D. Queen, Esquire, and Elizabeth Ellen Frasher, associate, with the national law firm of Ober, Kaler, Grimes & Shriver.

About the Authors

David D. Queen is a litigation partner with the firm of Ober, Kaler, Grimes & Shriver of Baltimore, New York and Washington, D.C. He specializes in designing corporate compliance plans, white collar criminal defense, and internal corporate investigations. Prior to entering private practice, Mr. Queen served as Deputy Assistant Secretary and Acting Assistant Secretary of the U.S. Department of the Treasury. He is the former United States Attorney for the Middle District of Pennsylvania, a former Assistant U.S. Attorney in Pennsylvania and Maryland, and a former Special Assistant U.S. Attorney for the District of Columbia.

Elizabeth Ellen Frasher is an associate in the Baltimore office of the law firm of Ober, Kaler, Grimes & Shriver. She specializes in designing and developing corporate compliance programs. Her practice also includes white collar criminal defense work and employment law.

CHAPTER 1

How the Sentencing Guidelines Apply to an Organization

Many organizations have policies, procedures and codes of ethics that they refer to as "compliance programs." These programs take many forms, varying greatly in scope and detail. Put such notions of corporate compliance out of your minds. Corporate compliance as used in this book is a term of art with a specific meaning, having fully entered the legal lexicon with the passage of The Sentencing Reform Act of 1984 (Title II of the Comprehensive Crime Control Act, 28 U.S.C. Sec. 994).

The Sentencing Reform Act was passed by a Congress that believed federal court sentences were applied unevenly, erratically and in an unpredictable manner. The act created the U.S. Sentencing Commission as an independent agency of the judicial branch. The commission has wide powers to establish sentencing policies and practices that must be followed by all federal judges when sentencing individuals and organizations. Among the stated purposes of the Act were uniformity and predictability in federal sentences.

The Federal Sentencing Guidelines went into effect in 1987. Initially, these guidelines applied only to individuals. Effective Nov. 1, 1991, however, the guidelines were expanded to include elaborate rules for the sentencing of organizations. Company officers and employees who are convicted of a federal crime are sentenced under the guidelines for individuals. The companies themselves are sentenced under the organizational guidelines.

An "organization" includes corporations, partnerships, associations, joint stock companies, unions, trusts, pension funds, unincorporated organizations, nonprofit organizations and even governmental bodies. In short, an organization is anything that is not an individual person (Sec. 8A1.1, Application Note l). In other words, your organization is included.

Of significance, the guidelines increased the number of individuals sentenced to jail, and the size of fines imposed on organizations. The former is very important for any counsel, whether representing the company or its employee. It is the latter, however, that is the subject of this book.

The organizational guidelines are contained in Sec. 8 of the Federal Sentencing Guidelines, and are reprinted in their entirety, along with application notes, as Appendix A at the end of this book.

The official introduction to Sec. 8 of the guidelines, which covers the sentencing of organizations, contains a succinct summary of its objective: "This chapter is designed so that sanctions imposed upon organizations and their agents, taken together, will provide just punishment, adequate deterrence, and incentives for organizations to maintain internal mechanisms for preventing, detecting and reporting criminal conduct."

True to its word, the Sentencing Commission created "incentives" for organizations to adopt such preventive measures. The most important incentive is the way in which corporate fines are calculated. Central to this calculation of every fine is the so-called "culpability score." According to the guidelines' introduction, "[c]ulpability generally will be determined by the steps taken by the organization prior to the offense to prevent and detect criminal conduct...." It is those "internal mechanisms" and "steps," which have become known as corporate compliance programs, that are the subject of this book.

The guidelines themselves are not statutes found in the U.S. Code. Rather, they are, as the name implies, guidelines, though they have the force and effect of law. Following each section of the guidelines' text, the Sentencing Commission has provided what it terms "Application Notes," as an aid to understanding the meaning of the guidelines. Throughout this book are references to specific sections of the organizational guidelines. They are set off in parentheses. For example, the definition of "high-level personnel" is found in Application Note 3(b), following Section 8A1.2. This would be cited as (Sec. 8A1.2, Application Note 3(b)).

Understanding the effect of the guidelines on an organization is the first step in answering the question raised in Chapter 2: Why does my organization need a compliance program?

CHAPTER 1 ADDITIONAL RESOURCES

Corporate Liability and Compliance

Gruner, *Corporate Crime and Sentencing*, The Michie Co., Charlottesville, Va. (1994).

A comprehensive, wide-ranging book on corporate criminality and liability, the organizational sentencing guidelines and compliance programs.

Webb, Molo and Hurst, "Understanding and Avoiding Corporate and Executive Criminal Liability," *49 The Business Lawyer 617* (February 1994).

This article addresses the steps a business organization can take to protect itself and its executives from criminal liability. It offers an in-depth discussion of the principles of corporate criminal liability, including liability of individuals directly associated with the corporation. It also discusses in detail the organizational sentencing guidelines and offers several sample calculations of sentences under the guidelines. Finally, the article discusses the importance and necessity of corporate compliance programs and the implementation of an effective compliance program.

Barr and Weinreich, "The Science of Compliance, U.S.-Style," *International Law Review* (September 1993).

This article discusses the dangers of ignoring the organizational sentencing guidelines, the benefits of a compliance program, and ways to structure, implement and enforce a compliance program.

Compliance Manual: Prevention of Corporate Liability, The Bureau of National Affairs Inc./American Corporate Counsel Assn., Vol. 1, Chapters 1 through 7 (1994), The Bureau of National Affairs Inc., 1231 25th Street N.W., Washington, D.C. 20037.

The BNA Compliance Manual is a guide to the establishment and operation of effective compliance programs to help insulate corporations and other organizations from criminal and civil liability. The manual is divided into several different chapters, each dealing with the different aspects of corporate compliance, beginning with compliance programs in the U.S. Sentencing Guidelines. The manual addresses environmental violations, health and safety violations, antitrust violations, government procurement laws, insider trading violations, bribery, fraud and false statements, and other aspects of federal criminal liability. This is an excellent resource for any organization attempting to design and implement an effective compliance program.

Prevention of Corporate Liability: Current Report, The Bureau of National Affairs Inc., 1231 25th Street N.W., Washington, D.C. 20037

This news bulletin is published monthly in conjunction with the BNA/ACCA *Compliance Manual: Prevention of Corporate Liability,* and is devoted to the latest developments in all aspects of corporate criminal liability and compliance programs.

Business Crimes Bulletin: Compliance in Litigation, Leader Publications, a division of New York Law Publishing Co.

This bulletin contains articles discussing the latest developments in corporate criminal liability and compliance programs.

The DOJ Alert, Prentice Hall Law and Business, 270 Sylvan Avenue, Inglewood Cliffs, N.J. 07632, (201) 894-5222.

This news bulletin discusses the latest developments in federal law and often is an excellent resource for developments in corporate criminal liability and compliance programs, including settlements with health care corporations and government-imposed compliance programs. It is a monthly bulletin on Department of Justice policies, procedures and tactics.

CHAPTER 2

Why Does My Organization Need a Compliance Program?

To understand why an organization needs a compliance program, one must first understand a typical organization's risk of prosecution in the modern world of federal criminal law.

Most organizations rightly see themselves as law-abiding. Therefore, any risk that the company might be charged with a crime seems slight, even remote. Most CEOs rightly believe theirs is not an outlaw company. With policies that prohibit violations of the law, they ask, "How can my organization be at risk?" The answer is simple: The government does not have to prove that breaking the law was corporate policy to indict and convict a company. It is enough that a crime occurred, even if it occurred at the lowest levels and was contrary to express corporate policy.

It is important that all business managers appreciate their organizations can be held criminally liable for the acts of employees, even if the employee was acting on his or her own and without the permission of upper management, so long as the employee was acting within the scope of his or her employment and to the benefit of the company.

As one legal scholar has noted:

"Establishing that an offense was committed willfully does not require a separate finding of corporate-level willfulness or fault. Rather, it is sufficient that an individual employee or agent acted with the necessary state of mind. Corporate liability in these situations is based on the attribution of employee actions and intent to corporate employers, not the fault of corporate managers...." Gruner, *Corporate Crime and Sentencing*, p. 199 (Michie, 1994).

Moreover, the organization can be held liable for the separate actions of several employees operating independent of one another, even if no single employee had the required intent to break the law. This "collective knowledge" applies when "the knowledge and conduct of multiple employees is attributed to a corporate principal and...is evaluated as if the collective knowledge and actions were undertaken by a single party." (See Gruner at p. 263).

As one court has observed:

> "[A] corporation cannot plead innocent by asserting that the information obtained by several employees was not acquired by any one individual employee who would then have comprehended its full import. Rather, the corporation is considered to have acquired the collective knowledge of its employees and is held responsible for their failure to act accordingly."

U.S. vs. T.I.M.E. - D.C. Inc., 381 F. Supp. 730, 738 (W.D. Va. 1974).

There is, however, some protection for organizations with stringent codes of conduct that are violated by employees. A "due diligence" defense has been recognized by some courts. Courts that recognize this defense, however, require a showing that the company's code of conduct has been effectively implemented and enforced. In other words, there must be an effective compliance program accompanying the rhetoric.

Thus, it is not enough for an organization to have a policy prohibiting wrongdoing or a simple ethics policy requiring conduct of the highest standards. Something more is necessary.

With an organization so easily at risk of prosecution, an effective compliance program is the best way to prevent unauthorized or unintended conduct and thereby reduce this risk. How this is accomplished will be explained in later chapters.

It is important to emphasize, however, that a compliance program must be "effective" to satisfy the guidelines. An "effective" corporate compliance program is "a program that has been reasonably designed, implemented and enforced so that it generally will be effective in preventing and detecting criminal conduct" (Sec. 8A1.2, Application Note 3(k)).

A company with a compliance program will enjoy several benefits, the most important being mandatory reductions in penalties imposed by a sentencing judge.

> "Under the guidelines, a company that adopts an effective program, turns itself in upon discovering a violation and cooperates with the prosecution, and has no involvement of high-level officials in the offense, may earn up to a 95% reduction in the penalty."

BNA/ACCA *Compliance Manual: Prevention of Corporate Liability*, Chapter 1, Sec. a-5d.

To appreciate the magnitude of these reductions in fines, it is first necessary to understand the mechanics of sentencing under the relatively new federal sentencing guidelines for organizations.

As noted in Chapter 1, a key purpose of the guidelines was to achieve equality and some degree of uniformity in sentencing. Consequently, a formulaic system was developed as part of a checklist that is used by the courts to calculate a numeric score. The organization's final "score" is then used in a sentencing table to determine the minimum and maximum allowable fine — the fine "range." It is within the "range" of minimum and maximum fines that the judge is permitted to exercise discretion in setting the final fine.

The following hypothetical will illustrate how a federal criminal sentence is computed under the guidelines. Let's begin with the Johnson Health Clinics Inc., a fictitious company with 200 employees that provides health care to Medicare patients. For several months, Johnson Health submitted claims using a procedure code that resulted in overpayments from the Medicare program totalling $1.6 million. After an investigation, federal prosecutors conclude that Johnson Health criminally violated the False Claims Act (18 U.S.C. Sec. 287).

Federal crimes are listed in the guidelines according to their statutory citations. A false claim (Sec. 287) is classified as a crime of fraud or deceit that has a score of six. This score is known as the "base offense level." The calculation of the base offense level is guided by Sec. 2F 1.1 (a)(b) of the guidelines, which is not included in the Appendix to this book. The base offense level is increased or decreased depending on the facts of the case, chief among them the loss to the crime's victim.

To calculate the loss to the victim in our hypothetical, the payments made by Medicare to Johnson Health would be aggregated. The "gain" to the organization is the total of all overpayments from Medicare. Using the appropriate table from the guidelines (Sec. 2F 1.1 (b)(1)), the loss of $1.6 million adds 12 points to the base offense level.

Here is the table from the guidelines:

Loss (Apply the Greatest)	**Increase in Level** (in points)
(A) $2,000 or less	no increase
(B) More than $2,000	add 1
(C) More than $5,000	add 2
(D) More than $10,000	add 3
(E) More than $20,000	add 4
(F) More than $40,000	add 5
(G) More than $70,000	add 6
(H) More than $120,000	add 7
(I) More than $200,000	add 8
(J) More than $350,000	add 9
(K) More than $500,000	add 10
(L) More than $800,000	add 11
(M) More than $1,500,000	add 12
(N) More than $2,500,000	add 13
(O) More than $5,000,000	add 14
(P) More than $10,000,000	add 15
(Q) More than $20,000,000	add 16
(R) More than $40,000,000	add 17
(S) More than $80,000,000	add 18

Obviously, the larger the "loss," the more points are added. The "base offense level" has now become the "offense level" with a score of 18 points, i.e., 6 points for the offense, plus 12 points for the amount of loss, as calculated from the above chart.

Two more points are added to the offense level if the offense required "more than minimal planning." Nearly all Medicare fraud schemes are seen by the government and courts as requiring more than "minimal planning."

Assuming no other aggravating circumstances, the final "offense level" is 20 points for our hypothetical crime, i.e., the total of 6 points for the "base offense," 12 points for the "loss," and 2 points for "more than minimal planning."

Next, the court must determine the "base fine" for the organization. The base fine is the greatest of (a) the gain to the organization from the crime, (b) the loss to the victim, or (c) an amount computed using the guidelines' fine table. The guideline fine is determined from the following table (Sec. 8C 2.4) that sets a dollar amount based on the final offense level score.

Offense Level	Amount
6 or less	$5,000
7	$7,500
8	$10,000
9	$15,000
10	$20,000
11	$30,000
12	$40,000
13	$60,000
14	$85,000
15	$125,000
16	$175,000
17	$250,000
18	$350,000
19	$500,000
20	$650,000
21	$910,000
22	$1,200,000
23	$1,600,000

Offense Level	Amount
24	$2,100,000
25	$2,800,000
26	$3,700,000
27	$4,800,000
28	$6,300,000
29	$8,100,000
30	$10,500,000
31	$13,500,000
32	$17,500,000
33	$22,000,000
34	$28,500,000
35	$36,000,000
36	$45,500,000
37	$57,500,000
38 or more	$72,500,000

Under this table, a score of 20 yields a fine of $650,000. Therefore, the largest of the three numbers (loss, gain or base fine) is clearly the loss figure — $1.6 million.

The court next determines what is known as the "culpability score" (Sec. 8C 2.5). This calculation automatically begins with five points. Points are added based on the size of the organization and the level of criminal involvement of upper management, among other factors. Points are added if as few as one person in a position of "substantial authority" participated in the crime, condoned it, or was willfully ignorant of the crime, or if "tolerance" of criminal conduct was pervasive within the company. The guidelines define "willful" ignorance as a failure "to investigate the possible occurence of unlawful conduct despite knowledge of circumstances that would lead a reasonable person to investigate whether unlawful conduct had occured" (Sec. 8A1.2, Application Note 3(j)). Such a company with any of the above characteristics and with 200 or more employees has 3 points added. More points are added for larger organizations. Assuming no other mitigating or aggravating facts, the culpability score in our hypothetical is 8.

The culpability score is then located on the "multiplier chart" (shown below and found at Sec. 8C 2.6) to determine the minimum and maximum multipliers.

Culpability Score	Minimum Multipler	Maximum Multiplier
10 or more	2.00	4.00
9	1.80	3.60
8	1.60	3.20
7	1.40	2.80
6	1.20	2.40
5	1.00	2.00
4	0.80	1.60
3	0.60	1.20
2	0.40	0.80
1	0.20	0.40
0 or less	0.05	0.02

With a score of 8, the minimum multiplier is 1.6 and maximum is 3.2. Those "multipliers" are then applied to the "base fine" to yield the minimum and maximum fines — the "range." The minimum fine in our hypothetical is therefore 1.6 times $1.6 million, or $2.56 million. The maximum fine is 3.2 times $1.6 million, or $5.12 million. The range within which the court must then impose its fine is therefore between $2.56 million and $5.12 million.

Now, assume the same fact situation with just one change; Johnson Health had an effective corporate compliance program.

At the point where the court calculates the culpability score, it is required to deduct 3 points if the organization had an effective corporate compliance program. Instead of a culpability score of 8, Johnson Health's score would be 5, which would reduce the fine range to between $1.6 million and $3.2 million.

The difference between the fine with a compliance program (ranging from $1.6 million to $3.2 million) and the fine without a program ($2.56 million to $5.12 million), could be as high as $3.52 million!

Another benefit of a corporate compliance program is that it creates a mechanism to detect violations before they get out of hand and often before they are discovered by government regulators. If your compliance program detects a violation of law, it is easier for your organization to self-report. If a company self-reports "prior to an imminent threat of disclosure or government investigation" and, within a "reasonably prompt" time of discovering the violation, cooperates with the federal government, and accepts responsibility, the court must deduct another 5 points from the culpability score. Coupled with the 3-point reduction for the existence of a compliance program, Johnson Health's culpability score would be zero if the company self-reported.

As the culpability score table shows, a culpability score of zero yields a minimum multiplier of .05 and a maximum multiplier of .20. Applied to the base fine of $1.6 million, the resulting fine range for Johnson Health would be between $80,000 and $320,000 if the company self-reported.

Thus, the difference between the minimum fine for Johnson Health with a compliance program that self-reports, and the maximum fine without a compliance program and without self-reporting, is $4.4 million! And remember, a criminal fine is not tax deductible! However, the costs of creating and operating a compliance program are.

The benefits of an effective compliance program go beyond reducing any fines from a violation. Among the less tangible benefits of a compliance program:

- It reduces the likelihood of a violation in the first place;
- It reduces the likelihood of civil liability;
- It gives management a different and generally more accurate view of the organization as it really is;
- It establishes a structure to disseminate legal and policy changes quickly and with the confidence that the communications will go beyond just the lawyers and top management;
- It establishes a structure to maximize the legally enforceable right of privacy under the attorney-client privilege; and

- It improves the speed and quality of responses to lawsuits, investigations and other emergencies that often occur with little or no warning.

How a compliance program achieves these additional benefits is explained in future chapters.

The preceding benefits alone should prompt an organization to adopt a corporate compliance program. But the reasons to adopt a program go beyond the positive benefits, which takes us to the issue raised in Chapter 3: What are the risks from not having a compliance program?

CHAPTER 2 ADDITIONAL RESOURCES

Benefits of a Corporate Compliance Program

Compliance Manual: Prevention of Corporate Liability, The Bureau of National Affairs Inc./American Corporate Counsel Assn., Chapter 1, Sec. A(5) (1994), The Bureau of National Affairs Inc., 1231 25th Street N.W., Washington, D.C. 20037.

Gruner, *Corporate Crime and Sentencing*, Chapter 14, The Michie Co., Charlottesville, Va. (1994).

A comprehensive, wide-ranging book on corporate criminality and liability, the organizational sentencing guidelines and compliance programs.

Barr and Weinreich, "The Science of Compliance, U.S.-Style," *International Law Review* (September 1993).

This article discusses the dangers of ignoring the organizational sentencing guidelines, the benefits of a compliance program, and ways to structure, implement and enforce a compliance program.

Webb, Molo, and Hurst, "Understanding and Avoiding Corporate and Executive Criminal Liability," *49 The Business Lawyer 617* (February 1994).

This article addresses the steps a business organization can take to protect itself and its executives from criminal liability. It offers an in-depth discussion of the principles of corporate criminal liability, including liability of individuals directly associated with the corporation. It also discusses in detail the organizational sentencing guidelines and offers several sample calculations of sentences under the guidelines. Finally, the article discusses the importance and necessity of corporate compliance programs and the implementation of an effective compliance program.

DeMuro and Roth, "Fraud and Abuse Compliance Programs: Their Time Has Come," *Health Care Financial Management* (March 1993).

Computing a Sentence Under the Guidelines

Bamberger and Gottlieb, *Practice Under the Federal Sentencing Guidelines,* Third Edition, Prentice Hall (1994).

A three-volume comprehensive source on the organizational sentencing guidelines and their legal impact.

Hutchinson and Yellen, *Federal Sentencing Law and Practice,* Second Edition, West Publishing (1994).

Compliance Manual: Prevention of Corporate Liability, The Bureau of National Affairs Inc./American Corporate Counsel Assn., Vol. 1, Chapters 1 through 7 (1994), The Bureau of National Affairs Inc., 1231 25th Street N.W., Washington, D.C. 20037.

Webb, Molo, and Hurst, "Understanding and Avoiding Corporate and Executive Criminal Liability," *49 The Business Lawyer 617, 641-654* (February 1994).

This article discusses in detail the organizational sentencing guidelines and offers several sample calculations of sentences under the guidelines.

CHAPTER 3

What Are the Risks from Not Having a Compliance Program?

In addition to the significant benefits from a compliance program described in the preceding chapter, there are risks to be considered for an organization that fails to adopt an effective compliance program.

Probation and Court-Imposed Programs

A company without a program that is convicted of a crime faces more than just a higher fine. It also faces a court-imposed compliance program. Under Sec. 8D1.1 of the guidelines, the court must impose probation of between one and five years if the organization has more than 50 employees and lacked an effective compliance program. Probation can include creation of a compliance program, which must be approved in advance by the court and which could include:

- Notification to employees and shareholders of the company's "criminal behavior";
- Periodic submissions to the court or a probation officer on the organization's financial condition, "results of business operations," and periodic "accounting for the disposition of all funds received";
- Periodic reports to the court or probation officer regarding the organization's program of operation, which must include (1) all information about investigations, litigation and administrative actions involving the organization, (2) regular and unan-

nounced visits to the organization by the probation officer, (3) examination of company books by the probation officer and experts hired by the court, (4) regular and periodic "interrogation[s] of knowledgeable individuals within the organizations"; and

- Payment by the organization of the costs for all of the above.

Government-Designed Programs

Even companies that are never charged with a crime can be subject to harsh programs. The Department of Justice has recently begun imposing compliance programs as part of out-of-court settlements. Two programs recently imposed by the government as part of publicly disclosed settlements have contained dramatically more onerous demands than are called for under the guidelines.

As part of an agreement with the government, a prominent health care products manufacturer was required to pay $61 million in fines and adopt a corporate compliance plan designed by the government. The government-imposed program went far beyond the minimum requirements of the guidelines and included such features as:

- Creation of a regulatory affairs committee of the board "composed entirely of outside directors" to which all compliance information must be directed;
- Review of all important legal issues by outside counsel;
- Use of an "independent outside consultant acceptable" to the Food and Drug Administration. The consultant must spend, at the government's discretion and the company's expense, up to six weeks a year making "unannounced inspections or audits." The audit results must be "simultaneously" provided to the company and the FDA; and
- Prompt reporting of all violations to the government, along with the results of any company investigation of the violations.

In another recent case, a company not only paid nearly $380 million in penalties and fines but was required to implement compliance procedures that included:

- Giving Department of Health and Human Services (HHS) employees the absolute right to examine virtually all company records, and the right to interview employees during business hours;
- The hiring of an independent accounting firm at company expense, whose compliance audit results must be reported to the government;
- Periodic review by an independent organization to determine the "medical necessity and quality of services rendered" by the company;
- The use of written contracts approved by outside counsel for important business relationships;
- A requirement that adherence to the compliance program be "an element" of every manager and supervisor performance evaluation;
- An annual compliance report to the government signed by the chairman of the board and general counsel, under penalty of the federal perjury laws, certifying the company's compliance with its legal duties;
- The retention of all documents pertinent to a determination about the company's compliance activities; and
- The right of the government to order the company to take additional compliance steps at a cost to the company of "up to $500,000" annually.

The above requirements are just some of the serious impositions placed on these companies by the government. As troubling as the requirements might be, a Justice Department spokesman said in a recent speech that future agreements and compliance programs will likely not be as lenient as those described above.

If there is a lesson from these two examples, it is that an organization is better off designing its own program before the government designs one for it.

Corporate Death Sentence

In extreme cases, such as where the organization is deemed to operate primarily by "criminal means" or by "criminal purposes," the fine "shall be set at an amount (subject to the statutory maximum) sufficient to divest the organization of all its net assets" (Sec. 8C1.1). The first so-called corporate death penalty was imposed in 1993. (See *DOJ Alert*, Vol. 3, No. 15, November 1993).

Medicare/Medicaid Exclusion

For a health care provider, there is a second danger from a conviction arising out of Medicare/Medicaid program fraud — exclusion from the Medicare and Medicaid programs (see 42 U.S.C. Sec. 1320 a-6). In the health industry, exclusion is tantamount to a corporate death penalty. The existence of a compliance program does not prevent exclusion, but it does reduce the risk of corporate conviction, which, in turn, reduces the chance of a mandatory exclusion.

Management Liability

Individuals have always been subject to fines and jail for their involvement in a crime. Individuals committing crimes on behalf of, or at the direction of, a company are no different. Indeed, in many health care criminal prosecutions, charges are brought against both the company and culpable employees. Most corporate officers and managers believe, however, that they are invulnerable to prosecution unless they personally participated in a crime or expressly ordered it to take place. That false assumption could prove costly to members of management involved in wrongdoing. The introduction to the organizational guidelines spells this out clearly:

"Organizations can act only through agents and, under federal criminal law, generally are vicariously liable for offenses committed by their agents. At the same time, individual agents are [also] responsible for their own criminal conduct. Federal prosecutions of organizations therefore frequently involve individual and organizational co-defendants. Convicted individual agents or organizations are sentenced in accordance with the guidelines and policy statements in the preceding chapters. [The organizational sentencing guidelines are]...designed so that the sanctions imposed upon organizations and their agents, taken together, will provide just punishment, adequate deterrence, and incentives for organizations to maintain internal mechanisms for preventing, detecting and reporting criminal conduct."

Individual officers, directors and employees have always been subject to prosecution for their personal criminal conduct. Increasingly, however, under a principle sometimes called the "responsible officer doctrine," high-ranking officers and upper management can be convicted, fined and even imprisoned for the criminal conduct of subordinate employees — even though the officer did not authorize the crime and had no actual knowledge of the criminal conduct.

One author put it succinctly when analyzing a key U.S. Supreme Court decision on the subject: "The government offered no proof that the company president had any knowledge of the facts revealing the offense or that he actively participated in it in any way. Nonetheless, the Supreme Court upheld the conviction on the basis that the executive was in general control over the day-to-day affairs of the company, including the illegal transactions." Gruner, *Corporate Crime and Sentencing*, p. 804 (Michie Co., 1994).

In a later case, the Supreme Court applied the responsible officer doctrine using this language:

"The principle [has] been...applied whether or not the crime required 'consciousness of wrongdoing,' and it [has] been applied not only to those corporate agents who themselves committed the criminal act, but also to those who by virtue of their managerial positions...could be deemed responsible for its commission...[T]he liability of managerial officers did not depend on their knowledge...or participation.... It was enough...that by virtue of the relationship he bore to the corporation [the manager] had the power to prevent the act...." *U.S. vs. Park*, 421 U.S. 658, 672 (1975).

Many of the cases of personal management liability for corporate employee actions have turned on evidence of the manager's indifference to his or her duty to supervise and prevent criminal conduct. The very existence of an effective corporate compliance program, supported and encouraged by upper management, is powerful evidence that the organization's officers took steps to "prevent" any criminal conduct.

Stockholder Lawsuits

Another risk to management and the board of directors that is often overlooked is civil litigation from disgruntled stockholders. Stockholder derivative suits come in all shapes and sizes. They are costly and embarrassing, and can result in huge civil judgments. What does a stockholder derivative suit have to do with the Federal Sentencing Guidelines? Management of a company that receives a dramatically higher criminal fine due to the absence of a compliance program may have to explain to its stockholders why it did not adopt a compliance program. The hypotheticals in Chapter 2 graphically illustrate the measurable difference in fines against companies with and without programs.

Officers and directors who reject the expense and effort of a program better be prepared to explain this decision to their stockholders if there is ever a corporate criminal conviction.

Counsel's Liability

No less a figure than a former U.S. attorney general has termed it "malpractice" for in-house counsel not to advise his/her corporation of the benefits of a corporate compliance program. For in-house counsel, this advice should not stop with notification to the next party in the chain of command, typically the CEO. Instead, counsel should take steps to ensure that the true client, the corporation, is notified directly. That means making sure the company's board has been briefed on the importance of a program and the risks of continuing to operate without one.

'Qui Tam' Lawsuits

The federal False Claims Act includes both criminal and civil penalties that are discussed later in this book. The Civil False Claims Act provides that anyone who presents a false or fraudulent claim to the government is liable for a civil penalty of at least $5,000 and as much as $10,000 per claim, plus treble damages. The statute was amended in 1986 to eliminate the need to prove that a defendant had a specific intent to defraud. 31 U.S.C. Sec. 3729(b)(3).

In 1994 alone, nearly $1.1 billion was collected under this statute. What is most ominous for health care providers is that use of the statute against them has dramatically increased. Even more potentially troublesome is that the act permits private citizens to initiate false claims actions in the name of the government — so called "qui tam" cases. The incentive for such private suits is a guaranteed bounty of between 15% and 25% of whatever is recovered, with the remainder going to the government. Of the nearly $1.1 billion recovered in 1994 under the Civil False Claims Act, almost $400 million was from private qui tam suits. The total bounty paid to those plaintiffs was nearly $70 million.

By far, the greatest number of qui tam plaintiffs are employees of the companies being sued. Thus, every one of your organization's employees should be considered a potential private attorney general.

Employees are inside the company daily, observing what is happening, what mistakes are being made, what corners are being cut. An effective compliance program that prevents violations of the False Claims Act deprives an employee of a basis upon which to sue. A program that fails to prevent, but at least detects, violations before they become immense is nearly as beneficial because it at least reduces the severity of the violations. Moreover, a company that discovers its own violation, self-reports, and cooperates earns a reduced penalty. 31 U.S.C. Sec. 3729(a)(C).

But there is an intangible benefit as well. Many qui tam plaintiffs are able to claim the moral high ground by asserting that their employers, if not outright criminal in their behavior, were indifferent to quality control. By establishing a compliance program with substance, that argument is taken away.

Another feature of many qui tam cases is that employees learn of, and even participate in, the wrongdoing for months or years before bringing their lawsuits — without first reporting to management. The compliance program should require that employees promptly report suspicious or illegal conduct to company management. In so doing, the company is forcing the employee to choose between expressly violating the compliance plan by concealing what he or she knows, or promptly reporting that knowledge to management.

If the employee chooses the former, the worker no longer is the "white knight," and can even be discharged for violating express company policy, something that is otherwise much more difficult under the so-called "whistle blower" statutes. If the employee chooses the latter option, the company can promptly halt the violations, take remedial steps, and perhaps self-report — all of which reduce exposure to monetary loss.

Presumably you now agree that your organization would benefit from a compliance program. If so, you are ready to ask the question answered in Chapter 4: What are the requirements of a corporate compliance program?

CHAPTER 3 ADDITIONAL RESOURCES

'Qui Tam' Suits

Brody, "Recent Developments in the Area of Qui Tam," *Federal Bar News and Journal*, Vol. 37, #9 (December 1990).

Court Imposed Programs

Compliance Manual: Prevention of Corporate Liability, The Bureau of National Affairs Inc./American Corporate Counsel Assn., Vol. 1, Chapter 1, Sec. A-5(e); Vol. 2, Appendix Business Ethics Codes, Document 19: Corporate Compliance Program, C. R. Bard, Inc., p. 1900:1 (1994), The Bureau of National Affairs Inc., 1231 25th Street N.W., Washington, D.C. 20037.

Bamberger and Gottlieb, *Practice Under the Federal Sentencing Guidelines*, Sec. 16(E) *et seq.*, Third Edition, Prentice Hall (1994).

Management Liability

Compliance Manual: Prevention of Corporate Liability, The Bureau of National Affairs Inc./American Corporate Counsel Assn., Vol. 1, Chapter 2 (1994), The Bureau of National Affairs Inc., 1231 25th Street N.W., Washington, D.C. 20037.

Gruner, *Corporate Crime and Sentencing*, Chapters 3, 4, 5 and 13. The Michie Co., Charlottesville, Va. (1994).

"U.S. Wins First Corporate Death Sentence," *The DOJ Alert*, Vol. 3, No. 15, Nov. 15, 1993, p. 5. Prentice Hall Law and Business, 270 Sylvan Ave., Inglewood Cliffs, N.J. 07632, (201) 894-5222.

Webb, Molo, and Hurst, "Understanding and Avoiding Corporate and Executive Criminal Liability," *49 The Business Lawyer 617, 627-630, 654-656* (February 1994).

CHAPTER 4

What Are the Requirements of a Compliance Program?

We previously discussed the many benefits of a corporate compliance program, from the difficult-to-measure benefits, such as reducing the risks of prosecution or civil suits, to the very tangible, such as guaranteed reductions in criminal fines.

To achieve those benefits, however, your organization must have more than just a document called "Corporate Compliance Program"; you must have an "effective" compliance program. The Sentencing Commission has provided a straightforward set of requirements that any program must satisfy to have it be declared "effective."

The previously quoted definition of an effective compliance program bears repetition: "An 'effective program to prevent and detect violations of law' means a program that has been reasonably designed, implemented and enforced so that it generally will be effective in preventing and detecting criminal conduct" (Sec. 8A1.2, Application Note 3(k)).

Fortunately, a program need not be foolproof. "Failure to prevent or detect [an]...offense, by itself, does not mean that the program was not effective" (Sec. 8A1.2, Application Note 3(k)).

The Application Notes provide a useful outline of what the Sentencing Commission declares are the "minimum" requirements:

"The hallmark of an effective program to prevent and detect violations of law is that the organization exercised due diligence in seeking to prevent and detect criminal conduct by its employees and other agents. Due diligence requires at a minimum that the organization must have taken the following types of steps:

Compliance Standards & Procedures

"(1) The organization must have established compliance standards and procedures to be followed by its employees and other agents that are reasonably capable of reducing the prospect of criminal conduct.

Oversight Responsibilities

"(2) Specific individual(s) within high-level personnel of the organization must have been assigned overall responsibility to oversee compliance with such standards and procedures.

"(3) The organization must have used due care not to delegate substantial discretionary authority to individuals whom the organization knew, or should have known through the exercise of due diligence, had a propensity to engage in illegal activities.

Employee Training

"(4) The organization must have taken steps to communicate effectively its standards and procedures to all employees and other agents, e.g., by requiring participation in training programs or by disseminating publications that explain in a practical manner what is required.

Monitoring & Auditing

"(5) The organization must have taken reasonable steps to achieve compliance with its standards, e.g., by utilizing monitoring and auditing systems reasonably designed to detect criminal conduct by its employees and other agents, and by having in place and publicizing a reporting system whereby employees and other agents could report criminal conduct by others within the organization without fear of retribution.

Enforcement & Discipline

"(6) The standards must have been consistently enforced through appropriate disciplinary mechanisms, including, as appropriate, discipline of individuals responsible for the failure to detect an offense. Adequate discipline of individuals responsible for an offense is a necessary component of enforcement; however, the form of discipline that will be appropriate will be case specific.

Response & Prevention

"(7) After an offense has been detected, the organization must have taken all reasonable steps to respond appropriately to the offense and to prevent further similar offenses — including any necessary modifications to its program to prevent and detect violations of law."

Your goal, therefore, is a program intended to prevent violations of law and, should prevention fail, to detect a violation. The three key steps are (1) design, (2) implementation, and (3) enforcement. By designing a program that incorporates the above seven steps, implementing the program fully and in conformity with these steps, and enforcing all of the program's requirements, you will assure your organization of having an "effective" program.

It is often said that the "devil is in the details." That expression applies to all three aspects of your corporate compliance program, from design to enforcement. But it is also true that a sound design will not save a poorly executed program. And a poorly designed program can never be effectively implemented. Care must be taken at each stage, beginning with the design of your program.

This takes us to the question answered in Chapter 5: Where do I begin the design of my organization's program?

CHAPTER 4 ADDITIONAL RESOURCES

Elements of a Compliance Program

Compliance Manual: Prevention of Corporate Liability, The Bureau of National Affairs Inc./American Corporate Counsel Assn., Vol. 1, Chapter 3 (1994), The Bureau of National Affairs Inc., 1231 25th Street N.W., Washington, D.C. 20037.

Webb, Molo, and Hurst, "Understanding and Avoiding Corporate and Executive Criminal Liability," *49 The Business Lawyer 617, 663-668* (February 1994).

Gruner, *Corporate Crime and Sentencing*, Chapter 14, The Michie Co., Charlottesville, Va. (1994).

Rakoff, Blumkin, and Sauber, *Corporate Sentencing Guidelines: Compliance and Mitigation*, Chapter 5, Law Journal Seminars — Press, 345 Park Avenue South, New York, N.Y. 10010 (1994).

CHAPTER 5

Where Do I Begin the Design of My Organization's Program?

The size of your organization affects the "degree of formality" of its compliance program. The larger the organization, the more formal the program (Sec. 8A1.2, Application Note 3(7)(i)). Although a written program is not expressly required under the guidelines, we view it as indispensable.

Among the first things your organization should do is adopt a resolution of the board of directors authorizing the creation of a corporate compliance program. If your organization has neither stockholders nor a board, then a simple letter to counsel from the majority stockholder(s) or CEO will suffice.

A board resolution has two important purposes. First, it documents the date on which your organization committed itself to creating a comprehensive compliance program. Thus, if your organization is implicated in wrongdoing before completion of the program, you can at least argue that your good intentions were not merely in response to a government investigation.

Second, and more important, the resolution is the first step in extending the attorney-client privilege to the entire process of compliance program design. The resolution should expressly identify the purpose of the legal representation as securing legal advice for use in creation and implementation of a corporate compliance program.

Our starting point for designing the substantive program has been provided for us by the guidelines' authors with the first of the seven elements of an effective program: "The organization must have established compliance standards and procedures to be followed by employees and other agents that are reasonably capable of reducing the prospect of criminal conduct" (Sec. 8A1.2, Application Note 3(k)(1)).

The design of the corporate compliance program must therefore begin with the creation of the standards you intend to apply to your company. After all, without standards, how can there be procedures? How will supervisors know what to do? What compliance program training will you give your employees, and how can you possibly expect to discipline wayward employees? Also, without standards, what will the auditors look for?

But what are compliance standards? They are more than a corporate code of ethics. The purpose of the program is to prevent and detect "criminal conduct." Remember too, the guidelines are applied by the federal courts. Thus, compliance standards are at the very least the legal requirements found in the federal criminal statutes and regulations that are applicable to your organization's business activities. Here too, the guidelines provide illustrations.

For example:

> "If an organization handles toxic substances, it must have established standards and procedures designed to ensure that those substances are properly handled at all times. If an organization employs sales personnel who have flexibility in setting prices, it must have established standards and procedures designed to prevent and detect price fixing. If an organization employs sales personnel who have flexibility to represent the material characteristics of a product, it must have established standards and procedures designed to prevent fraud" (Sec. 8A1.2, Application Note 3(k)(7)(ii)).

Based on your company's history and its routine business practices, the program must identify all applicable federal criminal statutes and regulations. These become the heart of your corporate compliance standards. A basic working list of federal criminal legal duties applicable to your organization should first be compiled. This and subsequent steps require the advice of counsel with knowledge of both your organization and the often subtle and complex health care statutes and regulations.

An off-the-shelf compliance plan is barely worth the paper it is written on. The same is true of using someone else's compliance plan. The end result will be like driving the proverbial square peg into a round hole — it won't fit. As a consequence, your organization will have a plan that will not work because it cannot work. And if it does not work in all seven areas, then you will have failed to create an "effective" compliance plan.

Therefore, an analysis of the organization's actual methods of doing business is crucial. This step is often called the pre-plan "legal audit." Compliance plan standards written without a legal audit will be of marginal value because standards are meaningless without procedures to implement them. Also, your organization's procedures will be effective in direct proportion to (a) their specificity, and (b) their relationship to your actual practices.

Chapter 6 deals with the mechanics of the important pre-program legal audit. The knowledge gained from that process is vital to assuring that counsel and company alike understand what is actually taking place inside the organization and what problems need correction. Knowledge gained from the pre-plan legal audit also helps assure that the standards set forth in the eventual program truly match the organization's needs.

Equally important is the advice of counsel who is expert in the application and enforcement of federal criminal laws. This expertise is necessary in part because the program may eventually be scrutinized by federal prosecutors and judges. The prosecutors will review your organization's conduct to determine whether it was reasonable from a law enforcement perspective and whether the program was correctly designed and implemented to prevent and detect criminal conduct. Prosecutors will not be satisfied if the organization merely met the civil standards set by the Department of Health and Human Services. Again, if the program fails to prevent a crime and your organization is indicted, the final and most important critics of your program will be the prosecutor and the judge.

Although the primary impetus for most organizations to create a compliance program is to avoid or reduce liability under federal law, state criminal laws and important civil liability issues can and should be addressed. These should be considered when first designing the compliance program.

Numerous health care-related statutes impose civil money penalties. As the name implies, they are penalties, meaning they are generally not tax deductible. But because they are civil, their imposition does not result in a criminal conviction. Therefore, the usual collateral consequences of a criminal conviction, such as mandatory exclusion from Medicare, do not occur.

Because violations of statutes can result in enormous civil money penalties, a review of civil statutes and their inclusion in a compliance audit and eventual plan are worthwhile. The guaranteed benefit of a reduced fine (Sec. 8C2.5(f)) is not available, however, in the civil penalty context.

Nevertheless, an effective compliance plan remains highly beneficial because it reduces the likelihood of both civil and criminal violations. One of the most frightening non-criminal threats is the Civil False Claims Act, 31 U.S.C. Sec. 3729, which carries penalties of at least $5,000 plus twice the value of each claim up to a maximum of $10,000 plus three times the value of each claim. A violation of that act requires "no proof of specific intent to defraud…." 31 U.S.C. Sec. 3729 (b)(3).

In addition, many states have standards that are different or more stringent than those imposed by the federal government. Therefore, your program should not be written in a vacuum that might result in inadvertent failure to comply with state statutes.

Also, important non-health care crimes often apply to a health care organization. For example, if your organization is a publicly traded corporation, numerous securities laws may apply, such as those prohibiting insider trading (15 U.S.C. Sec. 78j(b) and Rule 10b-5, 17 C.F.R. Sec. 240.10b-5). If your organization has overseas interests, the Foreign Corrupt Practices Act may apply (15 U.S.C. Sec. 78a, 78m, 78dd-1, 78dd-2 and 78ff). A frequently overlooked set of statutes are those prohibiting bribery and the improper giving of gratuities and gifts to government employees. A corporate policy addressing campaign contributions should also be considered to avoid inadvertent criminal violations of the many restrictions of the federal election laws.

Many corporate compliance programs neglect to include procedures to prevent the hiring of illegal aliens. Recent immigration laws carry large fines and even jail terms. Other important duties include compliance with tax laws, the Employee Retiree Income Security Act (ERISA), the Occupational Safety and Health Act (OSHA), and so on. Depending on the nature of your organization's activities identified during the legal audit, counsel will likely recommend adding or deleting various statutes and regulations.

The establishment of the organization's standards goes beyond compliance with criminal statutes and regulations, however. "An organization's failure to incorporate and follow applicable industry practice or the standards called for by any applicable governmental regulation weighs against a finding of an effective program to prevent and detect violations of law" (Sec. 8A1.2, Application Note 3(k)(7)(iii)).

Using traditionally civil regulations as a basis for prosecution is on the rise. The *DOJ Alert* reported the recent guilty plea of Ortho Pharmaceuticals that is instructive. Ortho agreed to pay $7.5 million and leave several individuals fully exposed for touting an acne drug as a wrinkle remover, something for which the drug was not approved. "If true, the claims would have been a regulatory crime," according to the *DOJ Alert*, Vol. 5, No. 4, March 6, 1995, p. 4. But as the *Alert* noted, there is an alarming trend.

"Retin-A may prove to be both safe and effective for wrinkles. But the lack of concrete economic or safety consequences is a distinction of diminishing significance to the government, where authorities are committed to the belief that subverting the regulatory structure can be as detrimental to real human victims, albeit indirectly, as organized crime," said the *DOJ Alert*.

Applicable regulations, even those without any criminal sanctions, must therefore be identified and included if their violation could be reasonably seen as having contributed to a violation of a criminal statute. Likewise, standards set by professional associations, trade groups and the like should be reviewed to determine if failure to adhere to them could increase the likelihood of a separate criminal violation.

In addition to the criminal statutes that apply to health care providers, there are numerous federal and state document retention statutes and regulations. The basic purpose of these rules is to require that documents important to government agencies are created and preserved for a specific time period so that they are available for review by investigators and auditors. Chapter 8 contains a discussion of the importance of including a comprehensive document system as part of your organization's compliance plan.

Ideally, there should be just one comprehensive pre-program audit. It should be carefully thought out in advance so that all relevant employees and managers are interviewed and all important documents are reviewed. Therefore, the precise document rules applicable to your organization should be identified and included in your listing of legal duties. These duties must be identified and understood before the pre-program audit begins.

Because documents play such a central role in nearly every health care provider's operation, their importance should be fully understood in advance. It stands to reason that if your organization is required to create and retain a certain type of document, the audit team should interview those responsible for doing both. The ability to intelligently question those employees will be severely impaired if the audit team does not understand these duties in advance.

Finally, we recommend adding to the legal duties list your organization's most important existing policies or rules that you anticipate will continue after adoption of the compliance program. This offers an opportunity to find out how well you have communicated your policies in the past and will give the employees a direct chance to make suggested changes for the future.

With a comprehensive list of the duties you believe are applicable to your organization, it is now time to design your pre-program legal audit, which takes us to the questions answered in Chapter 6: What is a legal audit and how is it conducted?

CHAPTER 5 ADDITIONAL RESOURCES

Designing a Program

Compliance Manual: Prevention of Corporate Liability, The Bureau of National Affairs Inc./American Corporate Counsel Assn., Vol. 1, Chapter 3, The Bureau of National Affairs Inc., 1231 25th Street N.W., Washington, D.C. 20037 (1994).

Document Retention

Rakoff, Blumkin and Sauber, *Corporate Sentencing Guidelines: Compliance and Mitigation*, Chapter 5, Law Journal Seminars - Press, 345 Park Avenue South, New York, N.Y. 10010 (1994).

Tomes, *Health Care Records Management, Disclosure and Retention: The Complete Legal Guide*, Health Care Financial Management Assn., Director, Corporate/Institutional Sales, Probus Publishing Co., (800) 998-4644 (1993).

Skupsky, *Records Retention Procedures*, Information Requirements Clearinghouse, (303) 691-3600 (1990).

CHAPTER 6

What Is a Legal Audit and How Is it Conducted?

In its simplest terms, a compliance program legal audit is (1) the procedure used to determine how effectively an organization is currently complying with its legal duties, and (2) the identification of those changes that will be needed to create and operate an effective compliance program. A closely related goal is to determine if there are other organizational activities that implicate legal duties not previously known to the organization. A pre-program legal audit has many of the characteristics of an internal investigation conducted by company counsel in reaction to suspected wrongdoing. The latter are reactive in nature and often follow an investigation directed against the organization by insurance company auditors or the Departments of Justice or Health and Human Services. Because the reactive and proactive approaches have some issues in common, we have included internal investigation resources in our bibliography at the end of this chapter.

Designing an Audit Plan

The first step is to design an audit plan. Remember, one of the goals is to find out how your organization really operates. The plan should (1) have a clearly defined scope, (2) identify the personnel who will conduct the audit, (3) identify the individuals to be interviewed and the documents to be reviewed, and (4) spell out the steps to ensure the process is protected by the attorney-client privilege and the attorney work product doctrine.

With these objectives in mind, counsel should take steps to:

- Ensure that someone from management authorized to make interim decisions is identified. The audit team, particularly if supervised by outside counsel, must have a single person to whom it can turn for prompt decisions or help. Unless that person is identified in advance, the speed of the process will be jeopardized;
- Spell out the lines of communication before the audit begins. The audit team will be under pressure to pass information to management almost from the beginning. Everyone who views the process as threatening or potentially punitive will want to be included in the information process. The audit team should know in advance that all information will be kept confidential and disclosed only when necessary on a need-to-know basis.

The Scope of the Audit

The scope of the audit will be influenced by two things: the organization's legal duties discussed in the previous chapter, and the wishes of the organization. The audit process should be as extensive as the intended compliance program. In addition to the organization's legal duties, the audit plan should identify all conduct, reports and the like that may bring the organization into contact with the federal government and the relevant state governments, if the program is to be truly comprehensive.

The audit plan should also identify all conduct, reports and the like that bring the organization into contact with non-government entities, such as insurance intermediaries, if any aspect of these relationships puts your organization at risk of violating the law.

Remember, the audit plan should be flexible enough that as the audit process goes forward, the team should be alert for information that might require a change in emphasis to be made, the addition of documents to be reviewed, and witnesses to be interviewed.

Who Will Conduct the Audit?

The composition of the audit team will be influenced by such issues as cost, organization size and the management-employee relationship. But nothing is more important than ensuring that the audit process accomplishes these two goals:

- Getting an accurate picture of the organization's operation; and
- Preserving the confidentiality of the information obtained.

Both goals are generally best served by an audit conducted by or at least supervised directly by counsel — preferably outside counsel. It is extremely risky to have non-lawyers conduct the audit, whether they be employees of the organization or an outside auditing firm. That's because a key goal of the audit is honest employee disclosure. If employees reveal past or ongoing wrongdoing to the auditors, the content of the disclosures can later be demanded by government investigators unless protected by the attorney-client privilege. Furthermore, employees might be less inclined to reveal information to non-lawyers.

Moreover, the information gathered by the audit team will have limited use unless eventually analyzed by counsel skilled in both health law and corporate criminal liability. If counsel will eventually review the information, it stands to reason that counsel may as well collect it.

In-house counsel often participates in the audit design and sometimes in the audit process itself. The inclusion of in-house counsel is sometimes necessitated by the need to reduce costs, include someone knowledgeable about the organization, or both. As long as in-house counsel's presence will not have a chilling effect on employees, his or her inclusion is not necessarily detrimental. However, outside counsel should make sure that in-house counsel has historically served as a legal advisor and not merely a corporate officer with a law degree.

Who Will Be Interviewed?

The persons to be interviewed and the documents to be reviewed should be identified before the audit process starts. Of course, the list may change as data is discovered along the way. Nevertheless, the audit team must initially identify the personnel at all levels who can best educate team members on the operations most affected by the compliance program's standards and procedures.

No employee is too high-ranking or too low-level to skip over. For example, in a company that submits Medicare claim forms directly to the intermediary, the employees who submit the forms should be talked to. The audit team should have a healthy skepticism toward an upper-management that says low-level employees "know the rules and are doing as they have been told." Experienced counsel rarely conduct an audit without turning up behavior that startles management. Consider interviewing former employees or even former members of upper-management. Time and distance have a way of improving insight and candor.

The persons interviewed should be selected for questioning based on their likely knowledge of such topics as (1) existing company policies on important issues, (2) the frequency of training on such issues, (3) unethical or illegal conduct, (4) violations of existing company policies, (5) whether workloads are unreasonably heavy or result in corner-cutting, and (5) recommendations for improvements in employee training, ethical standards and the like.

Don't Forget Your 'Agents!'

A careful review of the Federal Sentencing Commission's seven minimum requirements for compliance programs elements discussed in Chapter 4 reveals a clear call by the drafters of the guidelines for organizations to take into account "agents" with whom firms subcontract or to whom they delegate responsibilities. Three of the seven elements of an "effective" plan expressly refer to an organization's responsibility for its agents' conduct:

(1) The program's standards and procedures must be "followed by its...agents";

(2) Communication of the program's requirements and training requires the organization to "have taken steps to communicate effectively its standards and procedures to...agents"; and

(3) The monitoring and auditing procedures must be "reasonably designed to detect criminal conduct by...agents."

The guidelines broadly define "agent" as "any individual, including a director, an officer, an employee, or an independent contractor, authorized to act on behalf of the organization" (Sec. 8A1.2, Application Note 3(d)).

Therefore, the legal audit team should identify in advance those who would qualify as "agents," like medical waste haulers, independent contractor "employees," billing services, and sales representatives. Their interaction with the organization should be studied and, where possible, agents should be interviewed and their contracts with your organization should be reviewed to ensure the agents are fully complying with the law in all activities that might implicate your organization. Remember, the guidelines require that you not delegate responsibility to those with a "propensity" to violate the law. Your review of the agents should therefore include steps to determine if their past conduct resulted in any criminal violations or serious complaints to or by regulatory agencies.

Explaining the Audit

No pre-program legal audit can be both productive and a complete secret. Therefore, everyone involved should strive to make it a cooperative effort among counsel, management and employees. How the role of the legal auditors is explained to employees is therefore important to establishing a good working relationship between the auditors and workers. A good explanation will also go a long way toward employee acceptance of the eventual compliance program.

A straightforward, honest explanation, first from management, then from legal auditors, is recommended. Otherwise, rumors can spread rapidly and create the impression that the company is in trouble with the law, or perhaps that outside lawyers are coming in to look for ways to reduce staff or assign blame. Once these rumors start, they are difficult to stop. Therefore, care must be taken in preparing the initial explanation to employees.

What form this explanation takes (e.g., memo, letters, or meetings) will be determined by the size of the company, its locations, the educational makeup of the employees, and the organization's established method of communication. Some large companies prepare information videos that introduce the auditors and explain their purpose. Smaller organizations often hold personal meetings. Regardless of the approach, employees should be told that the process is part of the company's desire to be a good corporate citizen, minimize violations of the law, and take advantage of the benefits of a compliance program.

Interview Pitfalls

If properly prepared, the employees to be interviewed will presumably be cooperative, even enthusiastic. An employee who is forthcoming, however, presents both an opportunity and a risk. Such employees are often a wealth of information about corner-cutting, violations of company policy, and even past or current wrongdoing. Therein lies a twofold risk: (a) subsequent, unwanted release of this information to the government, and (b) the possibility that the treatment of such disclosures will lead to further ethical or legal problems.

First we turn to protecting the disclosures made during the legal audit. If a government agency later demands the legal audit results, your organization should be in a position to invoke the attorney-client privilege. Whether a communication or document is protected by the attorney-client privilege or the attorney work product doctrine is largely a factual determination that will ultimately be made by a court. Among the most important considerations for the court will be (1) the intent of the parties at the time the communication occurred, or at the time the document was created; (2) whether the information was provided by counsel or sought from counsel primarily for the purpose of obtaining legal advice as opposed to obtaining business advice; and (3) whether the subsequent behavior of those claiming the privilege was consistent with that intent, such as whether the advice was used for exercising legal rights and judgments, and whether the parties safeguarded the relevant document.

The first step in documenting the intent of the parties has already been taken: the creation of a board resolution or similar document. That document should state that the organization has hired a named law firm or designated in-house counsel to take all necessary steps to acquire information so the firm or in-house counsel can advise the organization on the creation of a corporate compliance program.

Next, as previously mentioned, those participating in the process should either be attorneys or under the supervision of attorneys. Third, all documents produced by counsel and those assisting counsel should be appropriately labeled, disseminated on a need-to-know basis only within the client organization, and be adequately safeguarded. Finally, interviews conducted by counsel should be structured to maximize the privilege. Techniques for accomplishing this are discussed later in this chapter.

Second is the issue of how to treat employee disclosures. In the compliance context, counsel often forget that the employee is not the client. A common scenario goes like this: Corporate counsel interviews an employee who discloses knowledge about wrongdoing or perhaps admits personal involvement. Thereafter, corporate counsel reports these disclosures to the board along with recommendations for putting an end to the unlawful conduct. The employee is disciplined or fired.

A significant body of case law has developed around lawsuits brought by employees against their employers and corporate counsel on this point. The most common lawsuits involve a claim of defamation against the lawyer and corporation and a claim that the employee was led to believe he or she enjoyed a personal attorney-client relationship with the corporate attorney.

Corporate counsel must carefully secure an employee's coop eration, but do so without misleading the employee on the important issue of attorney-client privilege. The employee should be told explicitly the purpose of the interview, who the interviewers are, and for whom they work (the corporation). The employee should also be told that an attorney-client relationship exists between the attorney and the employer — not the employee. The employee should also be informed that some or all of what is said during the interview may be protected by the attorney-client privilege, but that it is a privilege which belongs to the employer.

The final version of the employee interview notes should contain verification of what the employee was told in this regard. The following language is suggested:

> "Before the interview began, the witness was advised that we were acting in our capacity as counsel for [the organization]. The witness was fur-

> ther advised that information revealed to or by the witness during the interview would be in the witness' capacity as an employee and agent of the company. We further explained that all such information was therefore protected from disclosure under the attorney-client and attorney work product privileges which belong to [the organization]. The witness was also informed that the decision to invoke or waive the privilege rests exclusively with [the organization]. The witness acknowledged understanding the above and agreed to be bound by the privilege."

Even if the employee is fully advised of counsel's role, there remains the risk that a report by counsel to the organization could contain conclusions about the employee's conduct that the worker believes are defamatory. The substance of the law of defamation is far beyond the scope of this book. The materials listed at the end of this chapter, however, provide helpful guidance on the subject.

The objective for counsel is therefore threefold: (1) obtain employee cooperation; (2) do so while preserving the corporation's attorney-client privilege; and (3) avoid creating a risk of new litigation against the corporation. This again highlights the importance of using counsel experienced in performing internal investigations.

Documents Review as Part of Interview

We have already mentioned the importance of statutes and regulations that require the retention of certain documents. A complete list of such requirements applicable to your organization should be prepared in advance of the audit and used in the questioning of employees. If there are deficiencies in the organization's document retention system, the audit is the easiest place to discover this.

However, the document review portion of the audit must go beyond your organization's document retention duties to the content of the documents themselves. Whether or not covered by document retention requirements, documents play a central role in every health care organization. The "whys" and "hows" of their creation are just as important.

A well-thought-out document policy is central to any efficient compliance program. Few organizations have document systems that were designed with corporate compliance in mind. Hence, most organizations must make changes to their existing systems as part of their creation of a compliance program. It is self-evident, therefore, that a sound understanding of the existing document system should be part of the legal audit. Chapter 8 goes into greater detail on why a document system is important and the key considerations that should go into its design. Chapter 8 should be reviewed before the audit begins to identify additional areas for the audit.

Before employee interviews begin, the legal audit team should assemble representative documents from the organization's existing document system. Samples of the most important documents routinely created by the organization should be reviewed, especially those submitted to the government. Important documents received by your organization should also be included, where relevant.

The audit team should know in advance which employees create and review documents, and which employees determine the data included in documents. This process will also help identify employees for interviews.

Many of the questions that should be asked will be dictated by the organization's legal duties. For example, assume the organization generates medical waste. Employees should be asked about their training in the identification, handling and disposal of the waste along with their opinions about the reliability of any waste hauling subcontractors. In turn, the contract between your organization and the subcontractor should be reviewed, as should the subcontractor's practices.

For an organization that determines which CPT codes to assign to a service or what information should be included in a Medicare cost report, there should be a detailed examination of all procedures used to make those determinations. For example, the audit should identify those persons who prepare the reports or claims, how they review facts to determine what codes are used, what procedure they use to answer complicated or confusing questions, and how often the legal assumptions underlying their decision-making process are reviewed by counsel.

The interview questions to be asked should also be designed with an eye toward the final compliance program. The seven elements of an effective compliance program discussed in Chapter 4 should therefore be consulted in this process. Employees should be asked about past and current practices concerning organization standards, procedures, employee training and discipline, management oversight, monitoring and auditing, and complaints and wrongdoing handling. In short, the questions should solicit responses that indicate how current practices stack up against the standards your new compliance program will be required to meet.

Legally sufficient standards and procedures already in place should be identified for inclusion in the new program. Indeed, if the skeleton of a program already exists, your organization may be able to argue that a *de facto* program has been in existence for some time. This argument could prove beneficial should an investigation arise involving violations that pre-date your new program. More importantly, existing policies being considered for inclusion in the compliance program should be the basis for questions put to employees — questions such as whether these employees are even aware of the policy, whether the policy is accomplishing its goals, and how it can be improved.

The legal auditors should also be on the lookout for recent and even ongoing violations of law. Discovery of past violations will help determine what, if any, steps should be taken to proactively self-report before these violations are discovered by the government or insurance intermediaries, what measures must be enacted to end the violations, and what corrective measures should be taken.

At the close of the audit process, counsel should have:

- A solid working list of corporate legal duties applicable to the organization;
- An awareness of existing standards and procedures; and
- A familiarity with how the organization actually operates, where it is working well, and where the problems exist.

Counsel's Report and Recommendations

With this information, counsel is ready to make a report and recommendations to the organization. The content and formality of the report will depend on the specific circumstances.

Counsel's recommendations will depend heavily on what the legal audit has revealed. If ongoing or recent criminal activity has been unearthed, it clearly has to be dealt with, separately and distinct from the creation of the new compliance program. The handling of violations discovered in the legal audit should be undertaken only by skilled criminal counsel and is largely beyond the scope of this book. However, some helpful information can be found in Chapter 7 in the discussion of compliance program procedures for dealing with violations of law "detected" as part of the program.

CHAPTER 6 ADDITIONAL RESOURCES

Internal Audits and the Attorney-Client Privilege

Webb, Molo, and Hurst, "Understanding and Avoiding Corporate and Executive Criminal Liability," *49 The Business Lawyer 617* (February 1994).

Mulroy and Thessing, "Confidentiality Concerns in Internal Investigations," *Tort and Insurance Law Journal*, Vol. 25, No. 1 (Fall 1989).

diGenova and Riggs, "Protection of the Attorney-Client Privilege and Work Product After Martin Marietta: The Role of Outside Counsel in Internal Corporate Investigations," *Corporate Counsel's Quarterly*, Vol. 5, No. 4 (October 1989).

Faulkner, "Corporate Internal Investigations: A Checklist for Compliance," *Corporate Counsel's Quarterly*, Vol. 9, No. 1 (January 1993).

Webb, Tarun, and Molo, *Corporate Internal Investigations,* Chapters 9 and 11, Law Journal Seminars — Press, 345 Park Avenue South, New York, New York 10010 (1994).

Hallerud, "The Management of Criminal Investigations and Prosecutions, A Basic Outline for Corporate Counsel," prepared for the 1988 annual fall meeting of the American Bar Assn. Section on Litigation, Washington, D.C., October 20 and 22 (1988).

Barr and Weinreich, "The Science of Compliance, U.S.-Style," *International Law Review* (September 1993).

Defamation Concerns

Faulkner, "Corporate Internal Investigations: A Checklist for Compliance," *Corporate Counsel's Quarterly,* Vol. 9, No. 1 (January 1993).

Webb, Tarun, and Molo, *Corporate Internal Investigations,* Chapter 11, Law Journal Seminars — Press, 345 Park Avenue South, New York, New York 10010 (1994).

CHAPTER 7

What Must Be Included in the Compliance Program?

This chapter addresses those elements that must be included in any compliance program to be "effective" within the meaning of the guidelines.

If the legal audit has been thorough, the legal team should now have a solid knowledge of (1) the organization's existing standards and procedures, (2) its document system, (3) the organization's day-to-day operations, and (4) the organization's most important applicable legal duties. With that knowledge and the sentencing guidelines, the program can now be formulated.

Counsel and the organization must first agree on which current activities and policies must be discontinued and which are worth retaining. A note of caution: Lengthy policy and training manuals worth including in the compliance program, but too bulky to duplicate, are often incorporated by reference. This creates the risk that an incorporated policy included in a manual might be changed in the future, which could adversely affect the program's effectiveness. Care should therefore be exercised to ensure that all future revisions to such incorporated documents be approved in advance using a procedure set forth in the program.

As previously noted, many companies have seemingly stringent codes of ethics. But when carefully examined, they are usually conclusory and self-serving, lacking the kind of detail necessary to satisfy prosecutors or judges.

In fact, battles frequently erupt when counsel recommends to the organization's management specific procedures for implementing those standards in a formal compliance program. This is often the first time that management is faced with the difficult transition from its comfortable, but largely meaningless, code of ethics to standards that will almost certainly change the way the organization operates on a daily basis.

It is usually here that management first begins to calculate the cost of adopting standards that prohibit lucrative practices and/or procedures that require extra employee training and additional auditing requirements. In short, it is at this step that management often tries to pressure counsel to lower their sights.

No lawyer — least of all, in-house counsel — can force a client to follow advice. Counsel can merely advise against creating a compliance program that is flawed from the start. Remember: The program must be designed to operate as an "effective" program. Our earlier admonition bears repeating: A poorly designed program can never be effectively implemented.

When the organization and counsel are fully satisfied that the chosen standards are both commercially reasonable and satisfy at least the minimum legal requirements, the writing of the program can begin.

An important fact is often forgotten in drafting compliance programs: They cannot — indeed should not — be kept a secret. Most of the written program, if not all, will be distributed to employees at all levels of the organization. Therefore, the organization must be prepared to live with and adhere to whatever it puts on paper. Another equally important consideration is the audience to whom your program will be directed. In addition to the organization's employees, you should assume that investigators, prosecutors and judges will one day carefully scrutinize your program. Indeed, federal prosecutors increasingly are including demands for copies of corporate compliance programs in grand jury subpoenas. The HHS Inspector General's summonses are likely to start including similar demands.

You are now ready to begin drafting the compliance program. Some begin with introductory language setting forth the organization's intentions, a recital of the organization's long standing code of ethics, or a copy of the board's resolution adopting the program. However the program opens, its substantive portion should begin with a clear statement of the program's goal: creation of a compliance program that meets or exceeds the requirements of the Federal Sentencing Guidelines. Application Note 3(k) says it simply: the creation of a program to prevent and detect violations of law.

With the program's goals and objectives clearly stated, the program should address, in order, the seven minimum elements set out in Sec. 8A1.2, Application Note 3(k). For ease of understanding, we have divided below Application Note 3(k)(5) into two parts, resulting in eight substantive sections. We recommend a separate chapter in the plan to address each of the elements.

(1) Standards and Procedures

The substantive program should begin with the standards and procedures language of Application Note 3(k)(l) — the establishment of standards and procedures "reasonably capable of reducing the prospect of criminal conduct."

Thereafter, the standards the organization intends to adhere to should be enumerated. This is often the longest and most detailed portion of a compliance plan. A simple requirement that all employees obey the law will not suffice, but is merely the starting point. Each specific legal duty should be described with sufficient clarity that a reasonably intelligent employee can understand and follow it. For example, a specific law, regulation or insurance company policy could be paraphrased. The following policy prohibiting bribes and gratuities is an example:

> "***Bribes and Improper Payments.*** No employee may enter into any agreement or arrangement that calls for a commission, rebate, consultant or service agreement, bribe, kickback or otherwise, when such employee knows or should suspect from the surrounding circumstances or after a reasonable good faith inquiry, that the intent or probable result is to improperly reward, directly or indirectly:
>
> - Any employee or official or other representative of any government, governmental agency (including the military) or entity owned or controlled by a government;

- Any officer, director, employee, shareholder or other representative of a customer, supplier or other institution with which the organization has existing or prospective business relations; or
- Any officer, official, member or other representative of the union.

"Employees are prohibited from giving inducements to such individuals to take action favorable to the organization, whether relating to obtaining or retaining business or otherwise. The concept of an improper reward includes the giving of anything of value, not just money. For example, free or special price services or trips at company expense, without a proper business purpose, may constitute an improper payment just as readily as a cash payment. No action that would otherwise be suspect is permissible merely because it appears to be customary in a particular location or particular area of business activity.

"Small tips or gratuities given by employees of the organization to low-level, non-U.S. governmental personnel outside the U.S. for routine ministerial or clerical functions, for which the company is clearly entitled to give under local law are permitted if they are limited to customary amounts, are made only to facilitate proper performance of the officials' duties, and are properly recorded in the books and records of the organization. **Such payments shall not be made without the prior approval of the general counsel.**

"The practices of write-offs, discounting and forgiveness of debt are subject to interpretation as gifts, inducements or even bribes. The organization will establish a procedure to ensure that all such practices are based solely on justifiable business practices and are not utilized for improper purposes.

"Requests for special billing or payment procedures that suggest possible violations of law, such as evasion of income tax, currency exchange controls, or price or profit controls are contrary to the organization's policies, and no such billing or payment procedures shall be used. Such practices can also result in false, artificial or misleading entries in the books of the organization, which are strictly prohibited. Any questions regarding a particular practice should be addressed to the chief of compliance."

Where appropriate, following a recitation of the standard, procedures to assure adherence to that standard should be set forth. Remember that the program is an integrated document. Therefore, the monitoring and auditing section should address specific procedures to ensure that adherence to those procedures is covered in any audits.

(2) Oversight Responsibilities

The guidelines next require that "specific" individuals be assigned the duty of overseeing the compliance program. A general admonition to all employees will not suffice. The program must have a boss, who must be from "within high-level personnel."

The guidelines define "high level" as "individuals who have substantial control over the organization or who have a substantial role in the making of policy within the organization. The term includes a director; an executive officer; an individual in charge of a major business or functional unit such as sales, administration, or finance; and an individual with a substantial ownership interest" (Sec. 8A1.2, Application Note 3(b)).

The guidelines clearly will not permit the assignment of compliance supervision to a low-level functionary or a "fall guy." More than one "high-level" person can be assigned these duties, however. Sec. 2 of the program should therefore identify the compliance supervision individual(s). It is recommended that there be a single chief of corporate compliance. Only in the largest organizations is it likely that the position would be full-time and exclusive.

The chief of compliance should not only be given the power and resources to perform these important duties, but also the necessary time, especially in the early stages. These duties and powers should be clearly set forth in the program. Ambiguity in either area creates the risk that the compliance chief will fail to carry out his or her duties or that the compliance chief's ability to effectively "oversee" compliance will be undercut.

The listing of duties should not only be done with respect to the compliance chief. Other important positions should be identified and given enumerated duties. For example, if the organization has in-house counsel, counsel's duties involving compliance should be spelled out and counsel's relationship to the compliance chief should be described. The plan should spell out the following enumerated duties of counsel:

(1) To render all legal opinions necessary to the effective and prompt application of the plan. Where necessary, general counsel is authorized to secure the opinions of outside counsel, outside consultants and other experts.

(2) To carry out all duties set forth elsewhere in the compliance plan.

(3) To monitor all developments and changes in relevant state and federal statutes, regulations and court rulings that may affect the terms of the compliance plan.

(4) To promptly bring all such changes in the law to the attention of the chief of corporate compliance and to prepare proposed changes in the plan for submission to the chief of corporate compliance.

In the procedures section of the compliance program or in the section on monitoring, the program should expressly identify all activities that require advance review or approval by important officials, such as the CEO, chief of corporate compliance, and general counsel. In the case of either in-house or outside counsel, for example, if the organization has relationships reasonably likely to implicate the Medicare and Medicaid anti-kickback statute, the program should not only require adherence to the statute, but should require that (1) all such relationships be evidenced in a written contract; (2) those authorized to negotiate such contracts be identified in the compliance program; (3) the contracts be reviewed and approved in advance by counsel; (4) the contracts not contain an "evergreen" (self-renewing) clause; (5) the contracts have a specific termination date; and

(6) copies of all such contracts be retained in a central location, preferably the office of in-house counsel.

The compliance program should require the most sensitive or highest-risk contracts contain a clause that requires the signature of counsel or the chief of corporate compliance before the contract becomes effective. This provision reduces the risk in large organizations that a contract will be negotiated and put into effect before review by counsel. It will also make the auditing and monitoring functions, which are discussed later, much easier because the key contracts will be in one central location.

A key purpose of this section of your plan is twofold. First, it assures that important organizational functions are not delegated to potential law-breakers. Those in charge of hiring and firing, therefore, should be assigned explicit duties for screening applicants, where appropriate, for drug use, prior criminal records, reference checks and the like. This often-overlooked area is important because the guidelines require that important duties not be delegated to personnel "whom the organization knew, or should have known through the exercise of due diligence, had a propensity to engage in illegal activities" (Sec. 8A1.2, Application Note 3 (k)(3)). The contract review procedures previously discussed may even be advisable for a limited number of employment contracts to reduce the likelihood that important duties will be given to someone with a propensity to commit crimes.

The second purpose of this mechanism is to ensure that important duties under the program are not improperly delegated. To achieve this objective, the authority of key compliance program personnel to delegate duties must be specific. The following language is suggested:

> "Every assignment of responsibility and authority in this program is material. No oral delegation of responsibility or authority is permitted. Any delegation must be written and approved in advance by the chief of corporate compliance where practical. If the delegation is made by the chief of corporate compliance, prior approval must be obtained from the chief executive officer or general counsel, where practical. All delegations of responsibility and authority must be dated, signed by

the parties making and receiving the assignment, and copied promptly to the chief executive officer and general counsel."

(3) Employee Training

The third minimum step in the program requires that "[t]he organization must have taken steps to communicate effectively its standards and procedures to all employees and other agents" (Sec. 8A1.2, Application Note 3(k)(4)). The only suggestion offered in the guidelines as to how to meet this standard is that training may include "requiring participation in training programs or by disseminating publications that explain in a practical manner what is required."

Your final compliance program will be a written document. Much, if not all, can serve as the core of the written training materials. Employees take their cue from management and will adopt a level of enthusiasm toward the plan commensurate with what they see. Consequently, merely mailing the compliance program document to an employee, with the admonition that he or she read and obey it, is not enough. Face-to-face training, including lectures, videos or classes, is important.

First, such training greatly increases the probability that the employees will appreciate the importance of adherence to the program. Second, training will increase the probability they will actually absorb the material. Third, live training sessions will allow management to get employee reactions to the program and the training, and make adjustments to both, where needed. And fourth, such training will serve as later evidence to the government of your organization's level of commitment.

Section Three of the compliance program should therefore acknowledge the organization's training obligations, identify those responsible for the training, explicitly define what the training should include, and set deadlines for training of all existing employees. A procedure to train all new hires as a precondition for employment should be created as well.

Successful completion of employee training for new hires or within a specified time for existing employees should also be included in the program. The program should expressly forbid any employee, whether full or part-time, subcontracted or temporary, from acting on behalf of the organization without first having completed the employee screening and training process, unless written permission is obtained from the chief of corporate compliance.

In many large organizations, employee training might take months to complete. Indeed, just designing the training program could take weeks or months, depending on the diversity of employee duties and locations. With training, as with other parts of the program, formal adoption of the compliance program should not be held up until all details of the design are complete.

An appropriate compromise: Set a deadline for a specific individual to design a system for employee training with safeguards to assure that it is satisfactory.

At a minimum, the training should include education on all of the legal duties set forth in the "standards" section of your plan. If employee responsibilities vary greatly, training can be modified to reduce or expand the scope of training. We also strongly recommend establishing a system for responding to search warrants, attempts by agents to interview employees, etc. Employee training can be easily expanded to include education on this very important and often-overlooked area.

Finally, the compliance program should require periodic review of training procedures to ensure that the content of the materials is in accordance with current developments in the law. As previously noted, general counsel or outside counsel must regularly review legal developments that might affect the content of the program. The training section of the compliance program should specify that counsel, the chief of corporate compliance, and the training supervisor meet at least quarterly, monthly, or annually to accomplish this objective.

(4) Monitoring and Auditing

The fourth required element of an effective compliance program is that the organization "must have taken reasonable steps to achieve compliance with its standards" (Sec. 8A.1.2, Application Note 3(k)(5)). Interestingly, this language does not mandate an auditing or monitoring system. The Application Note, however, does give an example (not a definition) of "reasonable steps": "[U]tilizing monitoring and auditing systems reasonably designed to detect criminal conduct by its employees."

Note that the text of the Application Note calls for taking steps to "achieve compliance with [the organization's]... standards," while the example involves a system for affirmative crime detection. Nevertheless, most experts in the field have interpreted this section as requiring a structured audit system. The scope and complexity of the system will, of course, vary with the organization.

If the compliance program has comprehensive standards accompanied by procedures "reasonably capable of reducing the prospect of criminal conduct," then a monitoring system designed to "detect" crime would render Note 3(k)(5) redundant of Note 3(k)(1). We therefore interpret Application Note 3(k)(5) as requiring a system to monitor the operation of the compliance plan, with detection of crime as an important but secondary requirement.

Consequently, the monitoring and auditing system we recommend should review whether the compliance program is being followed — in short, whether the compliance program is serving its intended purpose. The procedures needed to audit the execution of the compliance program will be much different than the audit procedures in Note 3(k)(1) separately designed to otherwise detect crime. A good monitoring and auditing system can, of course, serve as one means to detect wrongdoing across the board.

In addition to avoiding possible duplication, this approach has two other benefits. First, it is less costly than a crime detection audit system. Second, it decreases the likelihood that the audit process will create non-privileged, damaging information.

The compliance program should therefore require creation of a system designed to audit the program's operational effectiveness. This can be accomplished in several ways. We recommend:

- The program describe a system to require spot checks of each of the procedures created as a result of Note 3(k)(l), to be performed by appropriate, specifically identified individuals. For example, if the program establishes procedures for medical waste disposal subcontractors, the audit should randomly review subcontractors to be sure they are covered by a current contract that meets program requirements;

- Selected individuals be required to verify at specified minimum intervals that other individuals have carried out their duties mandated under the program;
- Key duties assigned to personnel under the program include mandatory reviews by those individuals of the performance of other key program personnel; and
- If the organization employs certified public accounts, it consider adding an audit protocol to verify important compliance program tasks are being performed, such as required reports are prepared in a timely fashion, internal reviews are performed by supervisors, documentation supporting government claims are completed, employee training session are actually taking place, and employees are attending.

(6) Reporting System

The second half of Sec. 8A1.2's Application Note 3(k)(5) requires that "[t]he organization must have taken reasonable steps to achieve compliance with its standards... by having in place and publicizing a reporting system whereby employees and other agents could report criminal conduct by others within the organization without fear of retribution."

Thus, the program must create a reporting system and publicize it to employees and agents. Publicizing to employees is usually best achieved as part of the overall employee training program, because the employees must be taught more than just what telephone number to call. Many organizations also choose to post signs that summarize the reporting system in lunch rooms, locker rooms and key work areas.

The compliance program should mandate employees report conduct that a reasonable person would believe to be criminal. What constitutes a reportable event will, of course, be tied closely to the organization's policies spelled out in Section One of the plan and conveyed to employees as part of their compliance plan training.

If employees are required to report violations of the law or the program, then they must understand why, what the reporting system consists of, what will become of the information they provide, and what punishment they face if they fail to report.

The company must also do more than merely design a reporting system — often a so-called "hotline." It must also develop policies on what will be done with the information and how employees reporting the wrongdoing will be treated, and those policies must be communicated to the employees. By doing both, the organization can create confidence among employees that reported information is not being swept under the rug and that they will not be punished solely for making a report. The following is a suggested approach for a compliance program's handling of reports of wrongdoing:

> "The following shall be the policy and procedure for dealing with reports of wrongdoing.
>
> It shall be the policy of the company to take all reports of wrongdoing seriously. Reports of wrongdoing may be made orally, through the employee hotline, or in writing. Any such report must be directed to the chief of corporate compliance, who shall assure that the following steps are taken whenever possible:
>
> (1) A written record of the report shall be made using a form approved for use by general counsel or outside counsel. The chief of corporate compliance shall endeavor to obtain all information called for on the form;
>
> (2) No promises will be made to the party making the disclosure regarding his/her liability or what steps the company may take in response to the report of wrongdoing;
>
> (3) The chief of corporate compliance shall, upon completion of the reported wrongdoing, immediately contact general counsel to determine what steps will be taken;
>
> (4) General counsel and the chief of corporate compliance shall, at a minimum, determine whether the alleged wrongdoing is a violation of state or federal law, is a violation of the company compliance plan, poses a risk to the general public,

or otherwise puts the company at risk of economic injury or injury to reputation. Thereafter, the chief of corporate compliance and general counsel shall take action commensurate with the gravity of the allegation to determine if the allegation has a basis in fact, and what remedial action and/or punishment is to be imposed

If general counsel believes that the allegation, if true, would constitute a violation of either state or criminal law, he or she shall report that conclusion immediately to the chief executive officer and outside counsel;

(5) As part of general counsel's periodic reports to the board of directors, he or she shall include a report summarizing all allegations of wrongdoing, including the results of investigations and any subsequent punishments or remedial actions taken; and

(6) The company document retention program shall include provisions to assure that all records related to reports of wrongdoing are preserved in accordance with law and in a way that assures maximum protection under the attorney-client privilege and attorney work product doctrine."

The compliance program should also include procedures for the processing of the reports that preserve confidentiality and ensure that confirmed violations of law are dealt with in accordance with Application Note 3(k)(7) governing an organization's response to violations.

Whether the person actually taking the reports is the chief of corporate compliance, in-house counsel, a paralegal or an ombudsman, a written procedure for doing so should be part of the compliance program. Most systems for reporting wrongdoing consist of a so-called "hotline" and/or a specific individual to whom employees and agents can write.

Regardless of the form the reporting system takes, it should be simple and readily accessible to the employee, and should offer as much confidentiality and privacy as possible.

For purposes of simplicity, the organization should have a single telephone number, such as an 800 number, if the firm has employees in more than one telephone area code, and a single address for written reports. In-person reports should also be offered as an option. However, the latter should be discouraged in multi-site organizations because in-person reports tend to decentralize the system; centralization enhances uniformity of response and reduces the likelihood of unwanted disclosures.

To ensure accessibility, the hours of a hotline's operation are important. For most health care providers, a 24-hour hotline is unnecessary, unless the organization provides emergency services at unusual hours like a hospital does, or transports medical waste at unusual times of the day. Even an organization that is strictly 9-to-5, however, should offer some after-hours access, such as operating the hotline until 7:00 p.m. Offering optional ways to report wrongdoing also enhances flexibility.

The reporting system must also assure privacy and confidentiality. These two concepts are closely related, but different. Any reporting system should guarantee privacy to an employee who wishes to report wrongdoing. The system should offer some after-hours reporting so employees can call from home without fear of being overheard by fellow workers. Where face-to-face meetings are required — usually as a follow-up to the initial report — the system should offer after-hours meetings at neutral locations or even at the employee's home.

Confidentiality, on the other hand, is a much more difficult concept. As a matter of corporate policy, no program should promise complete confidentiality. Such a promise often cannot be kept and certainly cannot be made in advance of receiving the reported information. After all, the purpose of encouraging such reports is to act on those that have substance. Experienced litigators know that investigations of such reports can rarely be kept a secret, and that it is often easy for employees to discern the source of the report from the questions asked by investigators. Furthermore, in serious cases, depositions or testimony from the reporting employee may be essential. It is also important to remember that the organization may choose or be compelled to report a violation to the authorities, in which case the reporting employee's name will likely end up being disclosed.

A breached promise of confidentiality could also pit the employee against the organization and undermine the organization's credibility in the eyes of all employees. A promise of complete confidentiality may also compromise the company's position if it later concludes the reporting employee should be disciplined. We recommend a candid acknowledgment that complete confidentiality cannot be guaranteed.

Despite our call for flexibility in the reporting system, we strongly recommend a telephone reporting system for the following reasons:

- A phone system allows use of an optional caller ID system, through which a reporting employee who insists on withholding his or her name can be given a code number. This number helps the employee later prove that he or she actually made the report.
- A written report system makes it easier for the reporting employee to overlook or withhold important information. With a telephone system, the person taking the call can elicit important information to make sure the report is complete and includes as much information as possible to allow verification and further investigation. We also recommend that coded callers be told to call back on a specified future date using their code number so follow-up questions can be asked. No written system can accomplish this if the letter is anonymous.
- A telephone system ensures that the first written report of the alleged wrongdoing is prepared by a properly trained individual. Letters written by employees can contain inflammatory and conclusory information that is of little value and may potentially be very damaging. If, however, the organization chooses a written system, a basic form should be created and employees should be told to use that form exclusively for submitting reports to the organization.

Remember, a key feature of the guidelines is that employees and agents be permitted to report misconduct "without fear of retribution." The organization must do more than simply not retaliate against the reporting employee. Rather, it must create an atmosphere in which the employee is confident that he or she will not be the victim of retribution. We suggest the following language:

"It is the policy of [the organization] that no employee shall be punished solely on the basis that he or she reported what was reasonably believed to be an act of wrongdoing or a violation of this program or the company code of ethics.

However, an employee will be subject to disciplinary action if the company reasonably concludes that the report of wrongdoing was knowingly fabricated by the employee or was knowingly distorted, exaggerated or minimized to either injure someone else or to protect himself/herself or others.

In determining what, if any, disciplinary action may be taken against an employee, the company will take into account an employee's own admissions of wrongdoing; provided, however, that the reporting employee's conduct was not previously known to the company or its discovery was not imminent, and that the admission was complete and truthful. An employee whose report of misconduct contains admissions of personal wrongdoing will not, however, be guaranteed protection from disciplinary action. The weight to be given the self-confession will depend on all the facts known to the company at the time it makes its disciplinary decisions."

Who Should Handle the Reports?

By their very nature, reports of alleged wrongdoing are tricky. If true, they often implicate the organization and/or employees in criminal conduct.

First of all, these reports must be processed so as not to squelch one of the very objectives of the program: the detection of wrongdoing. A second, and nearly equally important concern is ensuring that the allegation is dealt with thoroughly and professionally. Third, the mechanism for handling reports should maximize the organization's rights to confidentiality. All three considerations suggest that someone associated with in-house counsel should be chiefly responsible for dealing with the initial report.

Whether in-house counsel should serve as the chief of corporate compliance is frequently a subject of intense debate. There is little debate, however, about the importance of counsel in the process of handling reports of wrongdoing. If not protected by the attorney-client privilege or attorney work product doctrine, all reports, investigations and remedial actions are subject to discovery in civil and criminal investigations. The organization may well choose to self-confess and make a full disclosure. As we have previously noted, however, self-confession should be an option unless mandated by statute, not a foregone conclusion. Even if the organization makes it a policy to report all violations of law to the authorities, the timing of those disclosures should, where possible, remain in the organization's hands.

We recommend that the initial reports of wrongdoing go directly to a legal counsel staff member likely to enjoy the protected attorney-client status. If the in-house counsel office is large enough, an associate general counsel should be designated to receive the reports. If the office is small, a paralegal or staff member trained in taking such reports should be used. In addition to increasing the likelihood of privilege, this approach helps to facilitate an expedited legal review of the report.

Organizations that do not have in-house counsel have a more difficult task of preserving the attorney-client privilege. The initial report will, of necessity, go to a non-lawyer. In such cases, we recommend that the chief of corporate compliance, or an assistant trained by outside counsel, take the information using the same procedures as those recommended for counsel. The forms used for initially recording the information should be clearly marked as being intended for direct transmission to counsel.

How Should the Reports Be Handled?

Reports of wrongdoing should be processed in a way that obtains the most complete information possible, permits a thorough investigation of the allegation if warranted, retains the organization's rights of confidentiality, and assures the greatest possible confidentiality for the person making the report.

The system should create enough of a paper trail to verify what and when the organization knew about the violation, as well as from whom it learned of the violation. We recommend a written intake form that is prominently marked "Attorney-Client Communication" and "Attorney Work Product." Those handling the reports should be trained on what to say and not say to those making the reports. Specifically these individuals should be instructed to (1) make no blanket promises of confidentiality; (2) make no predictions about how the information will be handled or what disciplinary action might be undertaken against the person reporting or others; and (3) explain to the caller the applicability of the attorney-client privilege to the information reported. In all three instances, the person taking the call should be required to read from a script to ensure uniformity of treatment. Some organizations print the canned recitations on the intake form with a notation that it was read to the caller.

We have already dealt with the importance of not promising the caller greater confidentiality than can be delivered. The other important issue is to ensure that the caller understands both the purpose of the call and the ownership of the information.

The entire process of employee reports of wrongdoing should be tied to obtaining legal advice rather than for making business decisions. As a consequence, the authors strongly believe that, properly structured, both the information received from an employee and the subsequent legal advice from counsel can be protected by the attorney-client privilege or work-product doctrine.

Every case turns on its own facts, of course, but any court review of a claim of privilege will begin with the intent and understanding of the parties at the time the information was exchanged. A claim of privilege will be enhanced if the parties treat the information as privileged from the start, mark all relevant documents accordingly, and create contemporaneous notations verifying that relationship.

Therefore, we recommend that employees making reports be reminded that they are calling in their capacity as employees of the organization, that they are speaking to a legal representative of the organization or a compliance official who will be immediately reviewing the information with counsel, and that the conversation is an attorney-client communication.

Remember the proviso that employees should be warned corporate counsel is not counsel for the employee but for the organization, and that the information may be disclosed to third parties at the sole discretion of the organization.

How the intake form is designed will vary significantly based on the organization's structure and primary purpose for doing business. The form should be designed, however, with the assistance of experienced counsel to ensure that the information obtained will be sufficient to permit an initial legal review to determine whether the allegation, if true, constitutes a crime or civil violation. The form must also elicit information sufficient to permit a follow-up investigation by representatives of the organization.

The intake form may be the only access the organization ever gets to the employee if the worker refuses to disclose his or her name and fails to call back in the future. Therefore, names, dates and the identity of witnesses with information should be included in the form.

The compliance program should also spell out procedures for how allegations of wrongdoing are handled. If allegations are first received by the chief of corporate compliance, the program should require that the report be forwarded immediately to counsel for review to determine whether it warrants further investigation, whether it requires immediate reporting to the authorities, or whether it can be classified as "without merit." Counsel's decision should be communicated to the chief of corporate compliance and, where appropriate, to the CEO or others within the organization. Routine decisions not to follow up on specific allegations should be included in a periodic report to management. Allegations that warrant further inquiry or emergency reporting to the authorities should be reported to management in accordance with a specific procedure. In no event should the allegations or their disposition be disclosed within the company except on a genuine need-to-know basis.

(7) Enforcement and Discipline

The guidelines require an enforcement system to put teeth into the compliance program. "The standards must have been consistently enforced through appropriate disciplinary mechanisms, including, as appropriate, discipline of individuals responsible for the failure to detect an offense" (Sec. 8A1.2, Application Note 3(k)(6)). No other instruction is provided except the admonition that the discipline be "adequate" and that the "form of the discipline that will be appropriate will be case-specific."

Key to understanding an organization's duties within this section are the words "consistently" and "mechanisms." The flexibility of allowing "case-specific" punishment does not mean that ad hoc discipline will suffice. A mechanism should be written into the compliance program to ensure that all employees and supervisors understand certain violations of the program will result in specific punishment.

Some commentators believe that adherence to the compliance program should be a specific criteria for promotions, bonuses and other employee "benefits." In other words, companies should offer an affirmative inducement for compliance rather than solely invoking negative punishment for non-compliance. If this carrot approach is used, it should be spelled out in the program and included in training.

Employees must be trained not only in their duties under the program, but be informed that the compliance plan creates a new class of acts and omissions that will require discipline of employees who fail to comply.

A frequently under-appreciated compliance program provision requires that employees be punished for a "failure to detect an offense." This provision goes beyond punishing only those employees who affirmatively break the law or expressly violate an important feature of the program. Rather, it also aims to punish employees who turn a blind eye to conduct that violates the program.

The compliance program should therefore require all employees and agents to report suspected violations of the law and breaches of the compliance program using the mechanisms in the reporting sections previously discussed. Included in the program's enumerated infractions should be punishment for employees who willfully fail to report wrongdoing. The following is suggested language to cover these requirements:

> "The Federal Sentencing Guidelines require that an "effective" compliance program include procedures to assure the discipline of employees "responsible for failure to detect" wrongdoing as well as for those who commit an offense or crime.

Therefore, all employees will be trained on the importance of adherence to the program and will be required to acknowledge that adherence to the program is a material condition of employment. Employees will be informed that failure to comply with the requirements of the program will result in discipline up to and including immediate discharge.

The company has a policy of progressive discipline for infractions committed by an employee, except where immediate termination is identified as the punishment. Whether the prohibited conduct constituted simple negligence, gross negligence or willfulness will be considered in determining and administering punishment.

The following list of employee infractions and violations apply to the company compliance program. They are a supplement to existing employee duties. Consistent with the Federal Sentencing Guidelines, the company will treat the listed infractions as follows:

Employee Action	Punishment
(1) Negligently providing incorrect information to the company or a government agency, consumer, insurer or the like.	First Offense: Second Offense: Third Offense:
(2) Willfully providing materially false information to the company or a government agency, customer, insurer or the like.	Termination
(3) Violation of any state or federal statute.	Termination
(4) Failure to report conduct by a company employee that a reasonable person should know is criminal.	Termination

Employee Action	Punishment
(5) Failure to report another employee's violations of any duties under this compliance program or reporting false or misleading information.	First Offense: Second Offense:
(6) Intentional misuse of the compliance hot line by knowingly and willfully providing false information to the chief of corporate compliance.	Termination
(7) Failure to detect conduct by an employee of the company that a reasonable person should know is criminal and reasonably could be expected to detect.	First Offense: Second Offense: Third Offense:
(8) Failure to take action as prescribed under the company compliance program or comply with any duties, express or implied, set forth in the program.	First Offense: Second Offense: Third Offense
(9) Engaging in any conduct prohibited in the employee handbook or that is considered unbecoming to a company employee.	First Offense: Second Offense: Third Offense:

If an employee has committed a violation of this program that would otherwise require termination, he or she may nevertheless be subject to a lesser punishment. Whether the employee is terminated will be influenced by (a) whether he or she promptly reported his/her own violation, (b) whether the report constitutes the company's first awareness of the violation and the employee's involvement, and (c) whether the employee cooperates fully in investigating and/or correcting the violation.

Whether the company eventually imposes a punishment less stringent than termination will be left to the sole discretion of the company.

The chief of corporate compliance together with the general counsel and the vice president for human resources shall within [___] days of the adoption of this compliance program by the board of directors, establish a uniform employee disciplinary procedure, which shall:

(1) Prohibit any waivers of disciplinary termination except by those persons expressly authorized to do so; and

(2) Prohibit any waivers of disciplinary actions prescribed in the employee handbook or compliance program except by those authorized to do so."

Any existing employee discipline plan must be carefully reviewed and revised where necessary to ensure that discipline resulting from a violation of the compliance plan is coordinated through the chief of corporate compliance. The reason for this should be obvious — any action serious enough to require discipline should be carefully reviewed by the chief of corporate compliance to determine if the program worked effectively and whether it needs any revision. Likewise, the employee's conduct may constitute a violation of law that could then trigger a duty to report the violation.

(8) Response and Prevention

The final mandatory element is found in Application Note 3(k)(7): "After an offense has been detected, the organization must have taken all reasonable steps to respond appropriately to the offense and to prevent further similar offenses — including any necessary modifications to its program to prevent and detect violations of law." This section contains three discrete parts: response, prevention and modification. This section of the compliance program must address all three.

The procedure for handling an unverified report of a violation is dealt with in the previous chapter of this book. The "Response and Prevention" section of a compliance program applies to the response to an "offense [that] has been detected." At this juncture, we are beyond an employee allegation of wrongdoing and into the realm of a completed and/or ongoing crime. We therefore assume that an completed inquiry by the chief of corporate compliance and counsel has determined that a crime has been committed.

It should go without saying that an organization failing to investigate a seemingly bona-fide report of wrongdoing or evidence unearthed through the monitoring and auditing procedures of the program has failed to "respond appropriately" to the violation. Remember, too, the guidelines' definition of "willful," which includes a "failure to investigate" (see Sec. 8C1.1). Therefore, the first milestone for an organization is its investigation and review of the earliest evidence of wrongdoing.

In Chapter 2 the mechanics of computing an organization's sentence was discussed. One of the key factors is the so-called "culpability score" (see Sec. 8C2.5. of the guidelines). The three-point deduction awarded to an organization with an effective compliance plan is not available, however, "if after becoming aware of an offense, the organization unreasonably delayed reporting the offense to appropriate governmental authorities" (Sec. 8C2.5(f)).

Application Note 10 to Sec. 8C2.5, says, however, that subsection (f) "contemplates…a reasonable period of time to conduct an internal investigation." Having a procedure in place that sets out rules for handling the reporting of violations and conducting an investigation has two substantive benefits: (1) it ensures that in the panic of the moment, important considerations are not overlooked; and (2) should the authorities independently discover the violation before the organization gets a chance to report it, the organization can more persuasively argue that it intended all along to make a full report, citing its compliance plan procedures as proof.

Second only to the criminal violation itself, the biggest mistake most organizations make is in their response to the violation. Ignoring a report of a violation potentially allows a criminal act to continue, thus increasing the number of violations and risking even greater penalties. Ignoring information that suggests a violation of law sets the stage later for punitive damage demands in civil cases or enhanced criminal fines. In some cases, there is a fine line between ignoring an offense and obstruction of justice.

Remember, the guidelines expressly assure that "[f]ailure to prevent or detect...[an] offense, by itself, does not mean that the program was not effective." When responding to a violation, the organization must neither panic nor cover up or turn a blind eye to an offense. Such reactions can cost the organization the right to call its program "effective," and thereby cause it to lose all of the sentencing benefits guaranteed under the guidelines. Covering up or ignoring an offense can even lead to additional crimes and charges. The best way to avoid aggravating the problem and to maximize the protections offered by the guidelines is to establish a simple checklist of things to do in the event a crime is detected.

The specific details of the discovered violation will play a large role in dictating the organization's "response." Therefore, after a violation is discovered, a program must ensure that nothing is done to compound the problem, that all legal obligations are fulfilled, and that the violation is turned to the organization's greatest advantage by preventing further violations and giving your organization the option to self-report before discovery by the government.

The policy of the organization should be clearly stated to require that all confirmed violations of law will be carefully reviewed using procedures designed to maximize the attorney-client privilege. This policy should require the chief of corporate compliance to consult with in-house counsel, or outside counsel where necessary, to determine whether disclosure is mandated by law or discretionary, and if the latter, whether and how authorities should be contacted.

If the organization engages in activities that pose a high risk of injury to persons, property or the environment, emergency procedures should be developed so employees know precisely when, where, and to whom they must report. In some cases, threats to public safety and the environment must be reported to the government. The compliance program's procedures must identify those employees responsible for notifying government agencies of a possible emergency, and provide for appropriate employee education and training. Such procedures will be the organization's first response to a violation, so the procedures should be prompt and complete.

Most crimes do not require self-reporting. For violations that do not require immediate reporting to the government, the response procedure should be more measured than for violations involving a public emergency or a statute requiring disclosure to the authorities. Here too, the precise response cannot be predicted in advance. However, a mechanism should be created to ensure that any decision on whether to self-report involves counsel and upper management and is made after a full review of the consequences of that decision.

If a decision is made to self-report, the compliance program should ensure that the organization gets the maximum credit for self-reporting. Therefore, the program should require that any report be "made under the direction" of the company and to the appropriate governmental authorities as defined in Sec. 8C2.5, Application Note 11. Also, the report should be "both timely and thorough" as defined in Sec. 8C2.5, Application Note 12. These two sections must be satisfied to gain the maximum sentencing credits, should the organization be prosecuted for the violation.

The Department of Justice recently announced its intention to develop a Voluntary Disclosure Program for the Department of Health and Human Services (*DOJ Alert* Vol. 4, No. 22, Dec. 19, 1994). The stated goal is a program similar to those covering the Department of Defense and the Justice Department's Environmental and Antitrust Divisions (See *Department of Justice Manual*, Vol. 4, Title 5, Section 11.301A).

The purpose of those programs is to establish clear criteria under which a company can know in advance what punishment it would receive. Under existing programs, companies that self-confess can even be assured of criminal amnesty in limited circumstances. One of the inducements under consideration for health care providers that self-confess would be a guarantee not to be excluded from Medicare.

The program is still in the talking stages. However, any chief of corporate compliance and counsel should remain current on developments in this area and ensure that its response to a discovered criminal violation takes into account the rules of any such future program.

Any procedure for responding to an allegation of wrongdoing must include at least an investigation and a report. If the investigation turns up compelling evidence of a crime, internally imposed employee punishment consistent with the program's procedures is essential, as is a revision to the compliance program to prevent future violations.

Whether the organization reports the violation to the authorities will depend on specific legal and practical considerations too numerous for discussion in this book. Either way, however, the paper trail created up to that point must be one you can live with. If a report is made to the authorities, then everything the organization has done up to that point will be scrutinized, including the conduct of counsel, the content of interview reports, punishment of miscreants, and so on.

If the decision is made to not report, there still remains a chance that the authorities will independently discover the wrongdoing. If they do, it will be especially important that the organization convince the prosecutor or judge that the decision to not self-report was, at a minimum, lawful.

The prevention requirement of Application Note 3(k)(7) calls for "reasonable steps" to prevent further similar offenses. No further guidance is provided. Prevention of further similar conduct should require that the chief of corporate compliance, in consultation with counsel, investigate to determine if the violation is ongoing. If it is, immediate steps must be taken to halt the behavior in question. Suspending or firing those responsible is one of the most obvious short-term solutions.

The compliance program should require that the report to the board on the violation contain both a description of what occurred and recommendations on what steps to take to prevent similar future conduct, which brings us to the final requirement of this Application Note — modification.

For a criminal violation to have occurred despite the existence of a compliance program, either the program failed to anticipate the offense altogether, or its procedures failed to prevent its occurrence. Whichever the case, the compliance program should be promptly and appropriately modified. The procedure for modifying the program should be spelled out to avoid an ill-considered change by someone not expressly authorized to make changes.

CHAPTER 7 ADDITIONAL RESOURCES

Compliance Program Design, Implementation and Operation

Compliance Manual: Prevention of Corporate Liability, The Bureau of National Affairs Inc./American Corporate Counsel Assn., Chapters 3, 4 and 5, (1994), The Bureau of National Affairs Inc., 1231 25th Street N.W., Washington, D.C. 20037.

Gruner, *Corporate Crime and Sentencing*, Chapters 3, 4, 5 and 13, The Michie Co., Charlottesville, Va. (1994).

Rakoff, Blumkin, and Sauber, *Corporate Sentencing Guidelines: Compliance and Mitigation*, Chapter 5, Law Journal Seminars Press, 345 Park Avenue South, New York, N.Y. 10010 (1994).

CHAPTER 8

The Role of a Document Policy in Compliance Programs

This chapter discusses one of the most important — and often ignored — aspects of a health care organization: its document system.

The importance of a system of documentation goes far beyond simply maintaining certain categories of records for specified periods of time. Documents, including computer tapes and other electronic "paper," are the heart and soul of most health care organizations, as they record treatment, establish contractual relationships, describe equipment specifications, etc. Also, documents are the medium by which claims and payments are made.

Still other documents are created that are perceived as exclusively internal but can prove pivotal in civil litigation, claims disputes, and audits, and, most important, in criminal investigations.

Documents never intended for disclosure outside the organization are subpoenaed in civil litigation as a matter of course in breach-of-contract disputes, malpractice cases and "qui tam" suits. Regulations give insurance intermediaries and the government a nearly absolute right to examine a provider's records (see 42 C.F.R. Sec. 1001.1301(a)(1)(iii) and (iv)). Generally, a provider has at least 24 hours within which to produce the requested records (Sec. 1001.1301(a)(3)), but provide them it must.

In criminal investigations, a federal grand jury subpoena reaches into an organization demanding all manner of notes, memos, appointment calendars, travel records and so on. A company without a carefully thought-out document system is not only hampered in its response to document demands, but is likely to discover that damaging documents were unnecessarily created, vital documentation was never created, or important documents were prematurely destroyed.

The core of any compliance plan is its standards. Procedures, training, discipline, auditing and response follow. It should be evident that none of these latter aspects of the compliance program will be fully effective if the organization lacks a coherent document system.

For many organizations, however, there is no "system" for handling documents. Instead, practices develop over the years, resulting in a hodge-podge that can hardly be called a "system" at all.

A document retention policy should at least meet the following standards:

- All records must be retained for at least the minimum period required by state or federal law or regulation.
- All records that may substantially affect the obligations of the company must be retained for a period of time that will reasonably ensure the availability of those records when needed.
- Adequate records must be developed and maintained to document the company's compliance with all relevant laws.
- Destruction of records must take place pursuant to a standard policy that has been developed for business reasons, to avoid allegations that the company deliberately destroyed records in anticipation of a specific problem.
- Any records-destruction procedure must have a mechanism that will ensure the procedure can be stopped to prevent the destruction of any appropriate records upon service of legal process for which those records might be relevant.
- The privacy and security of records MUST be appropriately assured.
- Records maintained on magnetic tape or other electronic data processing storage media must be covered by the compliance program.

What follows is a brief discussion of some of the more important health care records requirements.

Medicare requires providers to maintain and make available to the intermediary "records and documents [including medical records] necessary to ascertain information pertinent to the determination of the proper amount of [Medicare] payments due" (*Provider Reimbursement Manual*, PRM-1, Sec. 2304.1). In addition to this general requirement, Medicare designates several specific periods of retention. For instance, hospitals must retain clinical and other medical records relating to Medicare claims for at least five years after the month the Medicare cost report is filed with the intermediary (*Hospital Manual*, HIM-10, Secs. 413, 413.1). However, if the provider has reimbursement appeals for which the medical records might be relevant, the records for the relevant cost year should be retained until the appeal is finally resolved.

As a condition of Medicare participation, hospitals are required to retain medical records in their original or legally reproduced form for a period of at least five years (42 C.F.R. Sec. 482.24(b)(1)).

The Medicare Conditions of Participation also place various requirements on hospitals regarding the length of time records for specific services must be maintained. For instance, a hospital must maintain records of radiologic services, including copies of printouts and reports, films, scans and other image records for at least five years (42 C.F.R. Sec. 482.26(d)(2)). As for laboratory services, the conditions of participation require that hospitals must first ensure all such services provided to patients are performed in a facility certified under certain regulations (42 C.F.R. Sec. 482.27(a)). These regulations require that lab test requisitions or authorizations and records of patient testing, including an original report or an exact duplicate of each preliminary and final test report, must be retained for a minimum of two years after the date of reporting (42 C.F.R. Secs. 493.1105, 1007 and 1009). Immunohematology records, including reports, must be retained for no less than five years (42 C.F.R. Secs. 493.1107, 1109; 21 C.F.R. Part 606, Subpart 1). Pathology test reports must be retained for a period of at least 10 years after the date of reporting (42 C.F.R. Sec. 493.1109).

Medicare also has specific record retention requirements for:

- Long-term care facilities — a period required by state law, or, if there is no state requirement, for five years from the date of discharge for adults, and, for a minor, for three years after the resident reaches a legal age under state law (42 C.F.R. Sec. 483.75(1));
- Home health agencies — five years after the month the relevant cost report is filed (42 C.F.R. Sec. 484.38);
- Comprehensive outpatient rehabilitation facilities — five years after patient discharge (42 C.F.R. Sec. 485.60(c));
- Clinics and rehabilitation agencies that provide outpatient physical therapy and/or speech pathology services — a period determined by the state, or, if there is no state requirement, for five years after the date of discharge for adults and, for minors, three years after the patient becomes of age under state law or five years after discharge, whichever is longer (42 C.F.R. Sec. 405.1722(d)); and
- End-stage renal disease services — as required by state law, or, if there is no state requirement, for five years from the date of discharge or, in the case of a minor, three years after the patient becomes of age (42 C.F.R. Sec. 405.2140).

Methadone treatment programs must maintain records traceable to specific patients showing dates, quantity and batch or code marks of the drug dispensed for a period of three years from the date of dispensing (21 C.F.R. Sec. 291.505(d)(13)(ii)). Likewise, when narcotic drugs are administered for treatment of narcotic dependence for hospitalized patients, the hospital must maintain accurate records showing dates, quantity and batch or code marks for the drug used for at least three years (21 C.F.R. Sec. 291.505(f)(2)(u)).

Federal regulations protecting confidentiality of alcohol and drug abuse treatment records do not have specific general retention periods. However, the regulations require that the records be maintained in a secure room, locked file cabinet, safe or other similar container (42 C.F.R. Sec. 2.16). In addition, if a program discontinues operations or is acquired by another program, it must purge patient identifying records or destroy the records, unless the patient gives written consent to transfer the records or there is a legal requirement that the records be kept for a specific period. In such a case, the records are to be sealed and labeled with the name of the program and the citation to the court order or law requiring retention. Also, the records must be destroyed as soon as practical after the end of the required retention period (42 C.F.R. Sec. 2.19(a)).

State law may dictate specific medical record retention requirements. For example, Maryland law provides that, unless the patient is notified, a health care professional may not destroy an adult's medical records or laboratory or X-ray report until five years after the record or report is made (Maryland Health-General Article, Sec. 4-403(b)). In the case of a minor patient, a medical record, lab or X-ray report may not be destroyed until the patient attains the age of majority plus three years, or for four years after the record or report is made, whichever is later, unless the parent or guardian of the child is notified, or the minor patient is notified, if the care provided was care for which the minor is permitted to consent (Health-General Article, Sec. 4-403(c)).

State law related to Medicaid requirements may also dictate a specific retention period. For example, as a condition of participation in the Maryland Medicaid program, a provider must maintain adequate records for a minimum of six years (COMAR 10.09.36.03.) Although "adequate records" is not defined, the term is presumed to include medical records.

There are also statutes and regulations requiring privacy protection for certain classes of documents which may apply to documents created by your organization.

Creating a Document System

The responsibility for seeing that an appropriate records retention program is established should be assigned to a specific individual. As previously stated, however, there is more to caring for documents than merely retention. There should be a document "system."

What is a true document system? It is one with policies and procedures covering (1) creation, (2) distribution, (3) retention, (4) storage and retrieval, and (5) destruction of all documents.

Each of these areas must be addressed by policies that reflect the commercial realities and legal duties of the organization. Unless the final compliance plan contains express policies and procedures covering each of the five aspects of a document system, there is no system.

The biggest mistake an organization can make in this regard is to confuse a document retention policy with a comprehensive document system; they are not synonymous.

Put in its simplest terms, the policy behind the document system should be to create only those documents absolutely required by law and necessary to do business. Documents should be distributed to the smallest possible audience, with adequate security and retrieval safeguards. Finally, documents should be systematically destroyed at the earliest date permitted by law and by business needs.

Documents have two basic origins — internal and external — and separate approaches and policies are needed for each.

Document practices and policies typically cover those documents that are regularly or routinely created. The one-time document is not easy to pigeon hole in a document policy and must be dealt with differently.

All documents should be scrutinized with these questions in mind: Who created it and why? Where and how is it stored, and for how long? How long should it be retained? Is it subject to the attorney-client or attorney work product privilege? Would this document be relevant to any of the client's legal duties?

Externally Created Documents

Many documents sent to an organization must be retained, such as those evidencing a contractual relationship, proof of purchase, or proof of notice. Other documents, however, are of marginal long-term value. The key to reviewing externally created documents is to first determine which documents or types of documents are most likely to be regularly sent from an identified source, such as carrier bulletins, repeat invoices, shipping documents and the like. Once identified, these subcategories of documents should be examined to determine if the creator of the document has a clear pattern of identifying the recipient within the company. If there is more than one addressee, this should be reviewed to determine if such duplication is necessary and avoidable.

If there is only one addressee within the organization's structure, is the organization itself duplicating the document and distributing it within the company for review, action and storage? If so, the practice should be carefully reviewed.

That's because maintaining multiple copies of an externally created document is costly in terms of duplication and storage. Also, limiting a document's distribution also can reduce the scope of knowledge and access to the smallest universe possible. Limited circulation of documents also reduces the likelihood of disgruntled employees gaining access to the documents, and minimizes the probability that pirated copies will find their way outside the company.

To some degree, an organization can control many aspects of externally created documents. For example, if a supplier, agent or outside consultant regularly does business with the organization, the entity can often influence the subject matter and scope of the documents generated. Moreover, the organization can and should be certain that it, not the sender, decides who within the organization receives the documents.

Internally Created Documents

For internally created documents intended for internal consumption, the questions are often the same as for externally created documents, but with the important added question: Is this document necessary? If so, it should originate from or be addressed to the smallest necessary audience, and be afforded the maximum protection from scrutiny.

Another often-overlooked issue of importance is the content of the documents themselves. Documents that contain superfluous and potentially damaging information should be restructured accordingly.

Finally, there is the all-important issue of documents created by the organization for external consumption. These documents cannot be controlled once sent. Most important within this category are documents that must be submitted directly to a government agency. The federal false statement statute (18 U.S.C. Sec. 1001) and numerous industry-specific statutes carry severe penalties for providing false, fraudulent or materially misleading information. Even letters from the organization's counsel to another party's counsel are not protected unless pursuant to a joint defense agreement.

As previously stated, it should be the organization's policy to create only those documents that are (1) required to be created by law; (2) compelled by reason of business necessity; or (3) needed to obtain or follow legal advice. Documents not meeting these requirements should not be created.

It should also be the policy of the organization to distribute documents generated or received only to persons in and out of the organization on a need-to-know basis. Information copies ("FYI" copies) and the like should be discouraged. Documents should be distributed only to the addressee(s) and those expressly identified as requiring a copy. Any other copying, distribution or possession of documents should be prohibited.

It should also be the policy of the organization to retain documents created or generated only for the time required and in the manner required by law. Documents should be held beyond the legally required minimum time period only if required for reasons set forth in the organization's document retention plan.

CHAPTER 8 ADDITIONAL RESOURCES

Designing a Program

Compliance Manual: Prevention of Corporate Liability, The Bureau of National Affairs Inc./American Corporate Counsel Assn., Vol. 1, Chapter 3, The Bureau of National Affairs Inc., 1231 25th Street N.W., Washington, D.C., 20037 (1994).

Document Retention

Rakoff, Blumkin and Sauber, *Corporate Sentencing Guidelines: Compliance and Mitigation*, Chapter 5, Law Journal Seminars Press, 345 Park Avenue South, New York, N.Y., 10010 (1994).

Tomes, *Health Care Records Management, Disclosure and Retention: The Complete Legal Guide*, Health Care Financial Management Assn., Director, Corporate/Institutional Sales, Probus Publishing Co., (800) 998-4644 (1993).

Skupsky, *Records Retention Procedures*, Information Requirements Clearinghouse, (303) 691-3600 (1990).

APPENDIX

Federal Corporate Sentencing Guidelines

Index

United States Sentencing Commission Guidelines*

SENTENCING OF ORGANIZATIONS

Introductory Commentary

The guidelines and policy statements in this chapter apply when the convicted defendant is an organization. Organizations can act only through agents and, under federal criminal law, generally are vicariously liable for offenses committed by their agents. At the same time, individual agents are responsible for their own criminal conduct. Federal prosecutions of organizations therefore frequently involve individual and organizational codefendants. Convicted individual agents of organizations are sentenced in accordance with the guidelines and policy statements in the preceding chapters. This chapter is designed so that the sanctions imposed upon organizations and their agents, taken together, will provide just punishment, adequate deterrence, and incentives for organizations to maintain internal mechanisms for preventing, detecting, and reporting criminal conduct.

This chapter reflects the following general principles: First, the court must, whenever practicable, order the organization to remedy any harm caused by the offense. The resources expended to remedy the harm should not be viewed as punishment, but rather as a means of making victims whole for the harm caused. Second, if the organization operated primarily for a criminal purpose or primarily by criminal means, the fine should be set sufficiently high to divest the organization of all its assets. Third, the fine range for any other organization should be based on the seriousness of the offense and the culpability of the organization. The seriousness of the offense generally will be reflected by the highest of the pecuniary gain, the pecuniary loss, or the amount in a guideline offense level fine table. Culpability generally will be determined by the steps taken by the organization prior to the offense to prevent and detect criminal conduct, the level and extent of involvement in or tolerance of the offense by certain personnel, and the organization's actions after an offense has been committed. Fourth, probation is an appropriate sentence for an organizational defendant when needed to ensure that another sanction will be fully implemented, or to ensure that steps will be taken within the organization to reduce the likelihood of future criminal conduct.

Part A — General Application Principles

§ 8A 1.1. Applicability of Chapter Eight

This chapter applies to the sentencing of all organizations for felony and Class A misdemeanor offenses.

---

*56 Fed Reg 22762 (May 16, 1991).

1

Commentary

Application Notes

1. "Organization" means "a person other than an individual." 18 U.S.C. 18. The term includes corporations, partnerships, associations, joint-stock companies, unions, trusts, pension funds, unincorporated organizations, governments and political subdivisions thereof, and nonprofit organizations.

2. The fine guidelines in §§ 8C2.2 through 8C2.9 apply only to specified types of offenses. The other provisions of this chapter apply to the sentencing of all organizations for all felony and Class A misdemeanor offenses. For example, the restitution and probation provisions in parts B and D of this chapter apply to the sentencing of an organization, even if the fine guidelines in §§ 8C2.2 through 8C2.9 do not apply.

§ 8A 1.2. Application Instructions — Organizations

(a) Determine from Part B (Remedying Harm from Criminal Conduct) the sentencing requirements and options relating to restitution, remedial orders, community service, and notice to victims.

(b) Determine from Part C (Fines) the sentencing requirements and options relating to fines:

(1) If the organization operated primarily for a criminal purpose or primarily by criminal means, apply § 8C1.1 (Determining the Fine — Criminal Purpose Organizations).

(2) Otherwise, apply § 8C2.1 (Applicability of Fine Guidelines) to identify the counts for which the provisions of §§ 8C2.2 through 8C2.9 apply. For such counts:

(A) Refer to § 8C2.2 (Preliminary Determination of Inability to Pay Fine) to determine whether an abbreviated determination of the guideline fine range may be warranted.

(B) Apply § 8C2.3 (Offense Level) to determine the offense level from Chapter Two (Offense Conduct) and Chapter Three, Part D (Multiple Counts).

(C) Apply § 8C2.4 (Base Fine) to determine the base fine.

(D) Apply § 8C2.5 (Culpability Score) to determine the culpability score.

(E) Apply § 8C2.6 (Minimum and Maximum Multipliers) to determine the minimum and maximum multipliers corresponding to the culpability score.

2

(F) Apply § 8C2.7 (Guideline Fine Range — Organizations) to determine the minimum and maximum of the guideline fine range.

(G) Refer to § 8C2.8 (Determining the Fine Within the Range) to determine the amount of the fine within the applicable guideline range.

(H) Apply § 8C2.9 (Disgorgement) to determine whether an increase to the fine is required.

For any count or counts not covered under § 8C2.1 (Applicability of Fine Guidelines), apply § 8C2.10 (Determining the Fine for Other Counts).

(3) Apply the provisions relating to the implementation of the sentence of a fine in part C, subpart 3 (Implementing the Sentence of a Fine).

(4) For grounds for departure from the applicable guideline fine range, refer to part C, subpart 4 (Departures from the Guideline Fine Range).

(c) Determine from part D (Organizational Probation) the sentencing requirements and options relating to probation.

(d) Determine from Part E (Special Assessments, Forfeitures, and Costs) the sentencing requirements relating to special assessments, forfeitures, and costs.

Commentary

Application Notes

1. Determinations under this chapter are to be based upon the facts and information specified in the applicable guideline. Determinations that reference other chapters are to be made under the standards applicable to determinations under those chapters.

2. The definitions in the Commentary to § 1B1.1 (Application Instructions) and the guidelines and commentary in §§ 1B1.2 through 1B1.8 apply to determinations under this chapter unless otherwise specified. The adjustments in chapter Three, Parts A (Victim-Related Adjustments), B (Role in the Offense), C (Obstruction), and E (Acceptance of Responsibility) do not apply. The provisions of Chapter Six (Sentencing Procedures and Plea Agreements) apply to proceedings in which the defendant is an organization.

Guidelines and policy statements not referenced in this chapter, directly or indirectly, do not apply when the defendant is an organization; e.g., the policy statements in Chapter Seven (Violations of Probation and Supervised Release) do not apply to organizations.

3

3. The following are definitions of terms used frequently in this chapter:

(a) 'Offense' means the offense of conviction and all relevant conduct under § 1B1.3 (Relevant Conduct) unless a different meaning is specified or is otherwise clear from the context.

(b) 'High-level personnel of the organization' means individuals who have substantial control over the organization or who have a substantial role in the making of policy within the organization. The term includes: A director; an executive officer; an individual in charge of a major business or functional unit of the organization, such as sales, administration, or finance; and an individual with a substantial ownership interest. 'High-level personnel of a unit of the organization' is defined in the Commentary to § 8C2.5 (Culpability Score).

(c) 'Substantial authority personnel' means individuals who within the scope of their authority exercise a substantial measure of discretion in acting on behalf of an organization. The term includes high-level personnel, individuals who exercise substantial supervisory authority (e.g., a plant manager, a sales manager), and any other individuals who, although not a part of an organization's management, nevertheless exercise substantial discretion when acting within the scope of their authority (e.g., an individual with authority in an organization to negotiate or set price levels or an individual authorized to negotiate or approve significant contracts). Whether an individual falls within this category must be determined on a case-by-case basis.

(d) 'Agent' means any individual, including a director, an officer, an employee, or an independent contractor, authorized to act on behalf of the organization.

(e) An individual 'condoned' an offense if the individual knew of the offense and did not take reasonable steps to prevent or terminate the offense.

(f) 'Similar misconduct' means prior conduct that is similar in nature to the conduct underlying the instant offense, without regard to whether or not such conduct violated the same statutory provision. For example, prior Medicare fraud would be misconduct similar to an instant offense involving another type of fraud.

(g) 'Prior criminal adjudication' means conviction by trial, plea of guilty (including an Alford plea), or plea of nolo contendere.

(h) 'Pecuniary gain' is derived from 18 U.S.C. § 3571(d) and means the additional before-tax profit to the defendant resulting from the relevant conduct of the offense. Gain can result from either additional revenue or cost savings. For example, an offense involving odometer tampering can produce additional revenue. In such a case, the pecuniary gain is the additional revenue received because the automobiles appeared to have less mileage, i.e., the difference between the price received or expected for the automobiles with the apparent mileage and the fair market value of the automobiles with the actual mileage. An offense involving defense procurement fraud related to defective product testing can produce pecuniary gain resulting from cost savings. In such a case, the pecuniary gain is the amount saved because the product was not tested in the required manner.

(i) 'Pecuniary loss' is derived from 18 U.S.C. § 3571(d) and is equivalent to the term 'loss' as used in Chapter Two (Offense Conduct), except that pecuniary loss includes, for purposes of Chapter Eight, all damages from the offense that were caused intentionally, knowingly, or recklessly. See Commentary to §§ 2B1.1 (Larceny, Embezzlement, and Other Forms of Theft), 2F1.1 (Fraud and Deceit), and definitions of 'tax loss' in Chapter Two, Part T (Offenses Involving Taxation). For example, in a case of fraud upon the government involving product substitution or defective testing, loss may include (1) the government's costs of making substitute transactions and handling or disposing of the product delivered, or retrofitting the product so that it can be used for its intended purpose, and (2) the government s cost of rectifying the actual or potential disruption to government operations caused by the product substitution.

(j) An individual was 'willfully ignorant of the offense' if the individual did not investigate the possible occurrence of unlawful conduct despite knowledge of circumstances that would lead a reasonable person to investigate whether unlawful conduct had occurred.

(k) An "effective program to prevent and detect violations of law" means a program that has been reasonably designed, implemented, and enforced so that it generally will be effective in preventing and detecting criminal conduct. Failure to prevent or detect the instant offense, by itself, does not mean that the program was not effective. The hallmark of an effective program to prevent and detect violations of law is that the organization exercised due diligence in seeking to prevent and detect criminal conduct by its employees and other agents. Due diligence requires at a minimum that the organization must have taken the following types of steps:

(1) The organization must have established compliance standards and procedures to be followed by its employees and other agents that are reasonably capable of reducing the prospect of criminal conduct.

(2) Specific individual(s) within high-level personnel of the organization must have been assigned overall responsibility to oversee compliance with such standards and procedures.

(3) The organization must have used due care not to delegate substantial discretionary authority to individuals whom the organization knew, or should have known through the exercise of due diligence, had a propensity to engage in illegal activities.

(4) The organization must have taken steps to communicate effectively its standards and procedures to all employees and other agents, e.g., by

5

requiring participation in training programs or by disseminating publications that explain in a practical manner what is required.

(5) The organization must have taken reasonable steps to achieve compliance with its standards, e.g., by utilizing monitoring and auditing systems reasonably designed to detect criminal conduct by its employees and other agents and by having in place and publicizing a reporting system whereby employees and other agents could report criminal conduct by others within the organization without fear of retribution.

(6) The standards must have been consistently enforced through appropriate disciplinary mechanisms, including, as appropriate, discipline of individuals responsible for the failure to detect an offense. Adequate discipline of individuals responsible for an offense is a necessary component of enforcement; however, the discipline that will be appropriate will be case specific.

(7) After an offense has been detected, the organization must have taken all reasonable steps to respond appropriately to the offense and to prevent further similar offenses -- including any necessary modifications to its program to prevent and detect violations of law.

The precise actions necessary for an effective program to prevent and detect violations of law will depend upon a number of factors. Among the relevant factors are:

(i) Size of the organization -- The requisite degree of formality of a program to prevent and detect violations of law will vary with the size of the organizations: the larger the organization, the more formal the program typically should be. A larger organization generally should have established written policies defining the standards and procedures to be followed by its employees and other agents.

(ii) Likelihood that certain offenses may occur because of the nature of its business -- If because of the nature of an organization's business there is a substantial risk that certain types of offenses may occur, management must have taken steps to prevent and detect those types of offenses. For example, if an organization handles toxic substances, it must have established standards and procedures designed to ensure that those substances are properly handled at all times. If an organization employs sales personnel who have flexibility in setting prices, it must have established standards and procedures designed to prevent and detect price fixing. If an organization employs sales personnel who have flexibility to represent the material characteristics of a product, it must have established standards and procedures designed to prevent fraud.

(iii) Prior history of the organization -- An organization's prior history may indicate types of offenses that it should have taken actions to prevent. Recurrence of misconduct similar to that which an organization has previously committed casts doubt on whether it took all reasonable steps to prevent such misconduct.

An organization's failure to incorporate and follow applicable industry practice or the standards called for by any applicable governmental regulation weighs against a finding of an effective program to prevent and detect violations of law.

Part B — Remedying Harm from Criminal Conduct

Introductory Commentary

As a general principle, the court should require that the organization take all appropriate steps to provide compensation to victims and otherwise remedy the harm caused or threatened by the offense. A restitution order or an order of probation requiring restitution can be used to compensate identifiable victims of the offense. A remedial order or an order of probation requiring community service can be used to reduce or eliminate the harm threatened, or to repair the harm caused by the offense, when that harm or threatened harm would otherwise not be remedied. An order of notice to victims can be used to notify unidentified victims of the offense.

§ 8B1.1. Restitution — Organizations

(a) The court shall — (1) Enter a restitution order if such order is authorized under 18 U.S.C. §§ 3663-3664; or

(2) If a restitution order would be authorized under 18 U.S.C. §§ 3663-3664, except for the fact that the offense of conviction is not an offense set forth in title 18, United States Code, or 49 U.S.C. § 1472 (h), (i), (j), or sentence the organization to probation with a condition requiring restitution.

(b) Provided, that the provisions of subsection (a) do not apply when the organization has made full restitution, or to the extent the court determines that the complication and prolongation of the sentencing process resulting from the fashioning of a restitution requirement outweighs the need to provide restitution to any victims through the criminal process.

Commentary

Background: This guideline provides for restitution either as a sentence under 18 U.S.C. §§ 3663-3664 or as a condition of probation.

§ 8B1.2. Remedial Orders — Organizations (Policy Statement)

(a) To the extent not addressed under § 8B1.1 (Restitution — Organizations), a remedial order imposed as a condition of probation may require the organization to remedy the harm caused by the offense and to eliminate or reduce the risk that the instant offense will cause future harm.

(b) If the magnitude of expected future harm can be reasonably estimated, the court may require the organization to create a trust fund sufficient to address that expected harm.

Commentary

Background: The purposes of a remedial order are to remedy harm that has already occurred and to prevent future harm. A remedial order requiring corrective action by the organization may be necessary to prevent future injury from the instant offense, e.g., a product recall for a food and drug violation or a clean-up order for an environmental violation. In some cases in which a remedial order potentially may be appropriate, a governmental regulatory agency, e.g., the Environmental Protection Agency or the Food and Drug Administration, may have authority to order remedial measures. In such cases, a remedial order by the court may not be necessary. If a remedial order is entered, it should be coordinated with any administrative or civil actions taken by the appropriate governmental regulatory agency.

§ 8B1.3. Community Service — Organizations (Policy Statement)

Community service may be ordered as a condition of probation where such community service is reasonably designed to repair the harm caused by the offense.

Commentary

Background: An organization can perform community service only by employing its resources or paying its employees or others to do so. Consequently, an order that an organization perform community service is essentially an indirect monetary sanction, and therefore generally less desirable than a direct monetary sanction. However, where the convicted organization possesses knowledge, facilities, or skills that uniquely qualify it to repair damage caused by the offense, community service directed at repairing damage may provide an efficient means of remedying harm caused.

In the past, some forms of community service imposed on organizations have not been related to the purposes of sentencing. Requiring a defendant to endow a chair at a university or to contribute to a local charity would not be consistent with this section unless such community service provided a means for preventive or corrective action directly related to the offense and therefore served one of the purposes of sentencing set forth in 18 U.S.C. § 3553(a).

§ 8B1.4. Order of Notice to Victims — Organizations

Apply § 5F1.4 (Order of Notice to Victims).

Part C — Fines

I. Determining the Fine — Criminal Purpose Organizations

§ 8C1.1. Determining the Fine — Criminal Purpose Organizations

If, upon consideration of the nature and circumstances of the offense and the history and characteristics of the organization, the court determines that the organization operated primarily for a criminal purpose or primarily by criminal means, the fine shall be set at an amount (subject to the statutory maximum) sufficient to divest the organization of all its net assets. When this section applies, Subpart 2 (Determining the Fine — Other Organizations) and § 8C3.4 (Fines Paid by Owners of Closely-Held Organizations) do not apply.

Commentary

Application Notes

1. Net assets, as used in this section, means the assets remaining after payment of all legitimate claims against assets by known innocent bona fide creditors.

9

Background: This guideline addresses the case in which the court, based upon an examination of the nature and circumstances of the offense and the history and characteristics of the organization, determines that the organization was operated primarily for a criminal purpose (e.g., a front for a scheme that was designed to commit fraud; an organization established to participate in the illegal manufacture, importation, or distribution of a controlled substance) or operated primarily by criminal means (e.g., a hazardous waste disposal business that had no legitimate means of disposing of hazardous waste). In such a case, the fine shall be set at an amount sufficient to remove all of the organization's net assets. If the extent of the assets of the organization is unknown, the maximum fine authorized by statute should be imposed, absent innocent bona fide creditors.

2. Determining the Fine — Other Organizations

§ 8C2.1. Applicability of Fine Guidelines

The provisions of §§ 8C2.2 through 8C2.9 apply to each count for which the applicable guideline offense level is determined under:

(a) §§ 2B1.1, 2B1.2, 2B1.3, 2B2.3, 2B4.1, 2B5.3, 2B5.4, 2B6.1;
§§ 2C1.1, 2C1.2, 2C1.4, 2C1.6, 2C1.7;
§§ 2D1.7, 2D3.1, 2D3.2, 2D3.4;
§§ 2E3.1, 2E3.2, 2E3.3, 2E4.1, 2E5.1, 2E5.2, 2E5.3, 2E5.4, 2E5.5, 2E5.6;
§§ 2F1.1, 2F1.2;
§ 2G3.1;
§§ 2K1.1, 2K1.2, 2K2.1;
§ 2L1.1;
§ 2N3.1;
§ 2R1.1;
§§ 251.1, 251.2, 251.3, 251.4;
§§ 2T1.1, 2T1.2, 2T1.3, 2T1.4, 2T1.5, 2T1.6, 2T1.7, 2T1.8, 2T1.9, 2T2.1, 2T2.2, 2T3.1, 2T3.2; or

(b) §§ 2E1.1, 2X1.1, 2X2.1, 2X3.1, 2X4.1, with respect to cases in which the offense level for the underlying offense is determined under one of the guideline sections listed in subsection (a) above.

Commentary

Application Notes

1. If the Chapter Two offense guideline for a count is listed in subsection (a) or (b) above, and the applicable guideline results in the determination of the offense level by use of one of the listed guidelines, apply the provisions of §§ 8C2.2 through 8C2.9 to

10

that count. For example, §§ 8C2.2 through 8C2.9 apply to an offense under § 2K2.1 (an offense guideline listed in subsection (a)), unless the cross reference in that guideline requires the offense level to be determined under an offense guideline section not listed in subsection (a).

2. If the Chapter Two offense guideline for a count is not listed in subsection (a) or (b) above, but the applicable guideline results in the determination of the offense level by use of a listed guideline, apply the provisions of §§ 8C2.2 through 8C2.9 to that count. For example, where the conduct set forth in a count of conviction ordinarily referenced to § 2N2.1 (an offense guideline not listed in subsection (a)) establishes § 2F1.1 (Fraud and Deceit) as the applicable offense guideline (an offense guideline listed in subsection (a)), §§ 8C2.2 through 8C2.9 would apply because the actual offense level is determined under § 2F1.1 (Fraud and Deceit).

Background: The fine guidelines of this subpart apply only to offenses covered by the guideline sections set forth in subsection (a) above. For example, the provisions of §§ 8C2.2 through 8C2.9 do not apply to counts for which the applicable guideline offense level is determined under Chapter Two, Part Q (Offenses Involving the Environment). For such cases, § 8C2.10 (Determining the Fine for Other Counts) is applicable.

§ 8C2.2. Preliminary Determination of Inability to Pay Fine

(a) Where it is readily ascertainable that the organization cannot and is not likely to become able (even on an installment schedule) to pay restitution required under § 8B1.1 (Restitution — Organizations), a determination of the guideline fine range is unnecessary because, pursuant to § 8C3.3(a), no fine would be imposed.

(b) Where it is readily ascertainable through a preliminary determination of the minimum of the guideline fine range (see §§ 8C2.3 through 8C2.7) that the organization cannot and is not likely to become able (even on an installment schedule) to pay such minimum guideline fine, a further determination of the guideline fine range is unnecessary. Instead, the court may use the preliminary determination and impose the fine that would result from the application of§ 8C3.3 (Reduction of Fine Based on Inability to Pay).

Commentary

Application Notes

1. In a case of a determination under subsection (a), a statement that 'the guideline fine range was not determined because it is readily ascertainable that the defendant cannot and is not likely to become able to pay restitution' is recommended.

11

2. In a case of a determination under subsection (b), a statement that 'no precise determination of the guideline fine range is required because it is readily ascertainable that the defendant cannot and is not likely to become able to pay the minimum of the guideline fine range' is recommended.

Background: Many organizational defendants lack the ability to pay restitution. In addition, many organizational defendants who may be able to pay restitution lack the ability to pay the minimum fine called for by § 8C2.7(a). In such cases, a complete determination of the guideline fine range may be a needless exercise. This section provides for an abbreviated determination of the guideline fine range that can be applied where it is readily ascertainable that the fine within the guideline fine range determined under § 8C2.7 (Guideline Fine Range — Organizations) would be reduced under § 8C3.3 (Reduction of Fine Based on Inability to Pay).

§ 8C2.3. Offense Level

(a) For each count covered by § 8C2.1 (Applicability of Fine Guidelines), use the applicable Chapter Two guideline to determine the base offense level and apply, in the order listed, any appropriate adjustments contained in that guideline.

(b) Where there is more than one such count, apply Chapter Three, part D (Multiple Counts) to determine the combined offense level.

Commentary

Application Notes

1. In determining the offense level under this section, 'defendant,' as used in Chapter Two, includes any agent of the organization for whose conduct the organization is criminally responsible.

2. In determining the offense level under this section, apply the provisions of §§ 1B1.2 through 1B1.8. Do not apply the adjustments in Chapter Three, parts A (Victim-Related Adjustments), B (Role in the Offense), C (Obstruction), and E (Acceptance of Responsibility).

§ 8C2.4. Base Fine

(a) The base fine is the greatest of:

(1) The amount from the table in subsection (d) below corresponding to the offense level determined under § 8C2.3 (Offense Level); or

12

(2) The pecuniary gain to the organization from the offense; or

(3) The pecuniary loss from the offense caused by the organization, to the extent the loss was caused intentionally, knowingly, or recklessly.

(b) Provided, That if the applicable offense guideline in Chapter Two includes a special instruction for organizational fines, that special instruction shall be applied, as appropriate.

(c) Provided, further, That to the extent the calculation of either pecuniary gain or pecuniary loss would unduly complicate or prolong the sentencing process, that amount, i.e., gain or loss as appropriate, shall not be used for the determination of the base fine.

(d) Offense level fine Table

Offense level	Amount
6 or less	$ 5,000
7	7,500
8	10,000
9	15,000
10	20,000
11	30,000
12	40,000
13	60,000
14	85,000
15	125,000
16	175,000
17	250,000
18	350,000
19	500,000
20	650,000
21	910,000
22	1,200,000
23	1 600,000

13

Offense level	Amount
24	2,100,000
25	2,800,000
26	3,700,000
27	4 800,000
28	6,300,000
29	8,100,000
30	10,500,000
31	13,500,000
32	17,500,000
33	22,000,000
34	28,500,000
35	36,000,000
36	45,500,000
37	57,500,000
38 or more	72,500,000

Commentary

Application Notes

1. Pecuniary gain and pecuniary loss are defined in the Commentary to § 8A1.2 (Application Instructions — Organizations).

2. Under 18 U.S.C. 3571(d), the court is not required to calculate pecuniary loss or pecuniary gain to the extent that determination of loss or gain would unduly complicate or prolong the sentencing process. Nevertheless, the court may need to approximate loss in order to calculate offense levels under Chapter Two. See Commentary to § 2B1.I (Larceny, Embezzlement, and Other Forms of Theft). If loss is approximated for purposes of determining the applicable offense level, the court should use that approximation as the measure of pecuniary loss under this section.

3. In a case of an attempted offense or a conspiracy to commit an offense, pecuniary loss and pecuniary gain are to be determined in accordance with the principles stated in § 2X1.1 (Attempt, Solicitation, or Conspiracy).

4. In a case involving multiple participants (i.e., multiple organizations, or the organization and individual(s) unassociated with the organization), the applicable offense level is to be determined without regard to apportionment of the gain from or loss caused by the offense. See § 1B1.3 (Relevant Conduct). However, if the base fine is determined under subsections (a)(2) or (a)(3), the court may, as appropriate, apportion gain or loss considering the defendant's relative culpability and other pertinent factors.

5. Special instructions regarding the determination of the base fine are contained in: § 2B4.1 (Bribery in Procurement of Bank Loan and Other Commercial Bribery); § 2C1.1 (Offering, Giving, Soliciting, or Receiving a Bribe; Extortion Under Color of Official Right); § 2C1.2 (Offering, Giving, Soliciting, or Receiving a Gratuity); § 2E5.1 (Offering, Accepting, or Soliciting a Bribe or Gratuity Affecting the Operation of an Employee Welfare or Pension Benefit Plan); § 2R1.1 (Bid-Rigging, Price-Fixing or Market-Allocation Agreements Among Competitors); § 2S1.1 (Laundering of Monetary Instruments); § 2S1.2 (Engaging in Monetary Transactions in Property Derived from Specified Unlawful Activity); § 2S1.3 (Failure to Report Monetary Transactions; Structuring Transactions to Evade Reporting Requirements); and § 2S1.4 (Failure to File Currency and Monetary Instrument Report).

Background: Under this section, the base fine is determined in one of three ways: (1) the pecuniary gain to the organization from the offense; (2) the pecuniary loss caused by the organization; and (3) the amount, based on the offense level, from the table in subsection (d). In certain cases, special instructions for determining the loss, gain, or offense level amount apply. As a general rule, the base fine measures the seriousness of the offense. The determinants of the base fine are selected so that, in conjunction with the multipliers derived from the culpability score in § 8C2.5 (Culpability Score), they will result in guideline fine ranges appropriate to deter organizational criminal conduct and to provide incentives for organizations to maintain internal mechanisms for deterring, detecting, and reporting criminal conduct. In order to deter organizations from seeking to obtain financial reward through criminal conduct, this section provides that, when greatest, pecuniary gain to the organization is used to determine the base fine. In order to ensure that organizations will seek to prevent losses intentionally, knowingly, or recklessly caused by their agents, this section provides that, when greatest, pecuniary loss is used to determine the base fine in such circumstances.

Chapter Two provides special instructions for fines that include specific rules for determining the base fine in connection with certain types of offenses in which the calculation of loss or gain is difficult, e.g., price-fixing and money laundering. For these offenses, the special instructions tailor the base fine to circumstances that occur in connection with such offenses and that generally relate to the magnitude of loss or gain

15

resulting from such offenses. The offense level fine table in subsection (d) provides a residual or 'fall-back' method for setting the base fine.

§ 8C2.5. **Culpability Score**

(a) Start with 5 points and apply subsections (b) through (g) below.

(b) Involvement in or Tolerance of Criminal Activity

If more than one applies, use the greatest:

(1) If —

(A) The organization had 5,000 or more employees and

(i) An individual within high-level personnel of the organization participated in, condoned, or was willfully ignorant of the offense; or

(ii) Tolerance of the offense by substantial authority personnel was pervasive throughout the organization; or

(B) The unit of the organization within which the offense was committed had 5,000 or more employees and

(i) An individual within high-level personnel of the unit participated in, condoned, or was willfully ignorant of the offense; or

(ii) Tolerance of the offense by substantial authority personnel was pervasive throughout such unit, add 5 points; or

(2) If —

(A) The organization had 1,000 or more employees and

(i) An individual within high-level personnel of the organization participated in, condoned, or was willfully ignorant of the offense; or

(ii) Tolerance of the offense by substantial authority personnel was pervasive throughout the organization; or

(B) The unit of the organization within which the offense was committed had 1,000 or more employees and

16

(i) An individual within high-level personnel of the unit participated in, condoned, or was willfully ignorant of the offense; or

(ii) Tolerance of the offense by substantial authority personnel was pervasive throughout such unit,

Add 4 points; or

(3) If —

(A) The organization had 200 or more employees and

(i) An individual within high-level personnel of the organization participated in, condoned, or was willfully ignorant of the offense; or

(ii) Tolerance of the offense by substantial authority personnel was pervasive throughout the organization; or

(B) The unit of the organization within which the offense was committed had 200 or more employees and

(i) An individual within high-level personnel of the unit participated in, condoned, or was willfully ignorant of the offense; or

(ii) Tolerance of the offense by substantial authority personnel was pervasive throughout such unit,

Add 3 points; or

(4) If the organization had 50 or more employees and an individual within substantial authority personnel participated in, condoned, or was willfully ignorant of the offense, add 2 points; or

(5) If the organization had 10 or more employees and an individual within substantial authority personnel participated in, condoned, or was willfully ignorant of the offense, add 1 point.

(c) Prior History

If more than one applies, use the greater:

(1) If the organization (or separately-managed line of business) committed any part of the instant offense less than 10 years after (A) a criminal adjudication based on similar misconduct; or (B) civil or administrative adjudication(s) based on two or more separate instances of similar misconduct, add 1 point; or

(2) If the organization (or separately-managed line of business) committed any part of the instant offense less than 5 years after (A) a criminal adjudication based on similar misconduct; or (B) civil or administrative adjudication(s) based on two or more separate instances of similar misconduct, add 2 points.

(d) Violation of an Order

If more than one applies, use the greater:

(1) (A) If the commission of the instant offense violated a judicial order or injunction, other than a violation of a condition of probation; or (B) if the organization (or separately-managed line of business) violated a condition of probation by engaging in similar misconduct, i.e., misconduct similar to that for which it was placed on probation, add 2 points; or

(2) If the commission of the instant offense violated a condition of probation, add 1 point.

(e) Obstruction of Justice

If the organization willfully obstructed or impeded, attempted to obstruct or impede, or aided, abetted, or encouraged obstruction of justice during the investigation, prosecution, or sentencing of the instant offense, or, with knowledge thereof, failed to take reasonable steps to prevent such obstruction or impedance or attempted obstruction or impedance, add 3 points.

(f) Effective Program to Prevent and Detect Violations of Law

If the offense occurred despite an effective program to prevent and detect violations of law, subtract 3 points.

Provided, that this subsection does not apply if an individual within high-level personnel of the organization, a person within high-level personnel of the unit of the organization within which the offense was committed where the unit had 200 or more employees, or an individual responsible for the administration or enforcement of a program to prevent and detect violations of law participated in, condoned, or was willfully ignorant of the offense. Participation of an individual within substantial authority personnel in an offense results in a rebuttable presumption that the organization did not have an effective program to prevent and detect violations of law.

Provided, further, that this subsection does not apply if after becoming aware of an offense, the organization unreasonably delayed reporting the offense to appropriate governmental authorities.

(g) Self-Reporting, Cooperation, and Acceptance of Responsibility

18

If more than one applies, use the greatest:

(1) If the organization (A) Prior to an imminent threat of disclosure or government investigation; and (B) within a reasonably prompt time after becoming aware of the offense, reported the offense to appropriate governmental authorities, fully cooperated in the investigation, and clearly demonstrated recognition and affirmative acceptance of responsibility for its criminal conduct, subtract 5 points; or

(2) If the organization fully cooperated in the investigation and clearly demonstrated recognition and affirmative acceptance of responsibility for its criminal conduct, subtract 2 points; or

(3) If the organization clearly demonstrated recognition and affirmative acceptance of responsibility for its criminal conduct, subtract 1 point.

Commentary

Application Notes

1. 'Substantial authority personnel,' 'condoned,' 'willfully ignorant of the offense,' similar misconduct,' 'prior criminal adjudication,' and 'effective program to prevent and detect violations of law,' are defined in the Commentary to § 8A1 .2 (Application Instructions — Organizations).

2. For purposes of subsection (b), 'unit of the organization' means any reasonably distinct operational component of the organization. For example, a large organization may have several large units such as divisions or subsidiaries, as well as many smaller units such as specialized manufacturing, marketing, or accounting operations within these larger units. For purposes of this definition, all of these types of units are encompassed within the term 'unit of the organization.'

3. 'High-level personnel of the organization' is defined in the Commentary to § 8A1.2 (Application Instructions — Organizations). With respect to a unit with 200 or more employees, 'high-level personnel of a unit of the organization' means agents within the unit who set the policy for or control that unit. For example, if the managing agent of a unit with 200 employees participated in an offense, three points would be added under subsection (b)(3); if that organization had 1,000 employees and the managing agent of the unit with 200 employees were also within high-level personnel of the entire organization, four points (rather than three) would be added under subsection (b)(2).

4. Pervasiveness under subsection (b)will be case specific and depend on the number, and degree of responsibility, of individuals within substantial authority personnel who participated in, condoned, or were willfully ignorant of the offense. Fewer individuals need to be involved for a finding of pervasiveness if those individuals exercised a relatively

high degree of authority. Pervasiveness can occur either within an organization as a whole or within a unit of an organization. For example, if an offense were committed in an organization with 1,000 employees but the tolerance of the offense was pervasive only within a unit of the organization with 200 employees (and no high-level personnel of the organization participated in, condoned, or was willfully ignorant of the offense), three points would be added under subsection (b)(3). If, in the same organization, tolerance of the offense was pervasive throughout the organization as a whole, or an individual within high-level personnel of the organization participated in the offense, four points (rather than three) would be added under subsection (b)(2).

5. A 'separately-managed line of business,' as used in subsections (c) and (d), is a subpart of a for-profit organization that has its own management, has a high degree of autonomy from higher managerial authority, and maintains its own separate books of account. Corporate subsidiaries and divisions frequently are separately-managed lines of business. Under subsection (c), in determining the prior history of an organization with separately-managed lines of business, only the prior conduct or criminal record of the separately-managed line of business involved in the instant offense is to be used. Under subsection (d), in the context of an organization with separately-managed lines of business, in making the determination whether a violation of a condition of probation involved engaging in similar misconduct, only the prior misconduct of the separately-managed line of business involved in the instant offense is to be considered.

6. Under subsection (c), in determining the prior history of an organization or separately-managed line of business, the conduct of the underlying economic entity shall be considered without regard to its legal structure or ownership. For example, if two companies merged and became separate divisions and separately-managed lines of business within the merged company, each division would retain the prior history of its predecessor company. If a company reorganized and became a new legal entity, the new company would retain the prior history of the predecessor company. In contrast, if one company purchased the physical assets but not the ongoing business of another company, the prior history of the company selling the physical assets would not be transferred to the company purchasing the assets. However, if an organization is acquired by another organization in response to solicitations by appropriate federal government officials, the prior history of the acquired organization shall not be attributed to the acquiring organization.

7. Under subsections (c)(1)(B) and (c)(2)(B), the civil or administrative adjudication(s) must have occurred within the specified period (ten or five years) of the instant offense.

8. Adjust the culpability score for the factors listed in subsection (e) whether or not the offense guideline incorporates that factor, or that factor is inherent in the offense.

9. Subsection (e) applies where the obstruction is committed on behalf of the organization; it does not apply where an individual or individuals have attempted to conceal their misconduct from the organization.

20

10. The second proviso in subsection (f) contemplates that the organization will be allowed a reasonable period of time to conduct an internal investigation. In addition, no reporting is required by this proviso if the organization reasonably concluded, based on the information then available, that no offense had been committed.

11. 'Appropriate governmental authorities,' as used in subsections (f) and (g)(1), means the federal or state law enforcement, regulatory, or program officials having jurisdiction over such matter. To qualify for a reduction under subsection (g)(1), the report to appropriate governmental authorities must be made under the direction of the organization.

12. To qualify for a reduction under subsection (g)(1) or cooperation must be both timely and thorough. To be timely, the cooperation must begin essentially at the same time as the organization is officially notified of a criminal investigation. To be thorough, the cooperation should include the disclosure of all pertinent information known by the organization. A prime test of whether the organization has disclosed all pertinent information is whether the information is sufficient for law enforcement personnel to identify the nature and extent of the offense and the individual(s) responsible for the criminal conduct. However, the cooperation to be measured is the cooperation of the organization itself' not the cooperation of individuals within the organization. If' because of the lack of cooperation of particular individual(s), neither the organization nor law enforcement personnel are able to identify the culpable individual(s) within the organization despite the organization's efforts to cooperate fully, the organization may still be given credit for full cooperation.

13. Entry of a plea of guilty prior to the commencement of trial combined with truthful admission of involvement in the offense and related conduct ordinarily will constitute significant evidence of affirmative acceptance of responsibility under subsection (g), unless outweighed by conduct of the organization that is inconsistent with such acceptance of responsibility. This adjustment is not intended to apply to an organization that puts the government to its burden of proof at trial by denying the essential factual elements of guilt, is convicted, and only then admits guilt and expresses remorse. Conviction by trial, however, does not automatically preclude an organization from consideration for such a reduction. In rare situations, an organization may clearly demonstrate an acceptance of responsibility for its criminal conduct even though it exercises its constitutional right to a trial. This may occur, for example, where an organization goes to trial to assert and preserve issues that do not relate to factual guilt (e.g., to make a constitutional challenge to a statute or a challenge to the applicability of a statute to its conduct). In each such instance, however, a determination that an organization has accepted responsibility will be based primarily upon pretrial statements and conduct.

14. In making a determination with respect to subsection (g), the court may determine that the chief executive officer or highest ranking employee of an organization should appear at sentencing in order to signify that the organization has clearly demonstrated recognition and affirmative acceptance of responsibility.

21

Background: The increased culpability scores under subsection (b) are based on three interrelated principles. First, an organization is more culpable when individuals who manage the organization or who have substantial discretion in acting for the organization participate in, condone, or are willfully ignorant of criminal conduct. Second, as organizations become larger and their managements become more professional, participation in, condonation of' or willful ignorance of criminal conduct by such management is increasingly a breach of trust or abuse of position. Third, as organizations increase in size, the risk of criminal conduct beyond that reflected in the instant offense also increases whenever management's tolerance of that offense is pervasive. Because of the continuum of sizes of organizations and professionalization of management, subsection (b) gradually increases the culpability score based upon the size of the organization and the level and extent of the substantial authority personnel involvement.

§ 8C2.6 Minimum and Maximum Multipliers

Using the culpability score from § 8C2.5 (Culpability Score) and applying any applicable special instruction for fines in Chapter Two, determine the applicable minimum and maximum fine multipliers from the table below.

Culpability score multiplier multiplier
10 or more 2.00 4.00

Culpability score	Minimum multiplier	Maximum multiplier
10 or more	2.00	4.00
9	1.80	3.60
8	1.60	3.20
7	1.40	2.80
6	1.20	2.40
5	1.00	2.00
4	0.80	1.60
3	0.60	1.20
2	0.40	0.80
1	0.20	0.40
0 or less	0.05	0.20

22

Commentary

Application Note

1. A special instruction for fines in § 2R1.1 (Bid-Rigging, Price-Fixing or Market-Allocation Agreements Among Competitors) sets a floor for minimum and naximum multipliers in cases covered by that guideline.

8C2.7. Guideline Fine Range — Organizations

(a) The minimum of the guideline fine range is determined by multiplying the ase fine determined under § 8C2.4 (Base Fine) by the applicable minimum multiplier etermined under § 8C2.6 (Minimum and Maximum Multipliers).

(b) The maximum of the guideline fine range is determined by multiplying the ase fine determined under § 8C2.4 (Base Fine) by the applicable maximum multiplier etermined under § 8C2.6 (Minimum and Maximum Multipliers).

8C2.8. Determining the Fine Within the Range (Policy Statement)

(a) In determining the amount of the fine within the applicable guideline range, e court should consider:

(1) The need for the sentence to reflect the seriousness of the offense, romote respect for the law, provide just punishment, afford adequate deterrence, and rotect the public from further crimes of the organization;

(2) The organization's role in the offense;

(3) Any collateral consequences of conviction, including civil obligations ising from the organization's conduct;

(4) Any nonpecuniary loss caused or threatened by the offense;

(5) Whether the offense involved a vulnerable victim;

(6) Any prior criminal record of an individual within high-level personnel the organization or high-level personnel of a unit of the organization who participated , condoned, or was willfully ignorant of the criminal conduct;

(7) Any prior civil or criminal misconduct by the organization other than at counted under § 8C2.5(c);

23

(8) Any culpability score under § 8C2.5 (Culpability Score) higher than 10 or lower than 0;

(9) Partial but incomplete satisfaction of the conditions for one or more of the mitigating or aggravating factors set forth in § 8C2.5 (Culpability Score); and

(10) Any factor listed in 18 U.S.C. 3572(a).

(b) In addition, the court may consider the relative importance of any factor used to determine the range, including the pecuniary loss caused by the offense, the pecuniary gain from the offense, any specific offense characteristic used to determine the offense level, and any aggravating or mitigating factor used to determine the culpability score.

Commentary

Application Notes

1. Subsection (a)(2) provides that the court, in setting the fine within the guideline fine range, should consider the organization's role in the offense. This consideration is particularly appropriate if the guideline fine range does not take the organization's role in the offense into account. For example, the guideline fine range in an antitrust case does not take into consideration whether the organization was an organizer or leader of the conspiracy. A higher fine within the guideline fine range ordinarily will be appropriate for an organization that takes a leading role in such an offense.

2. Subsection (a) (3) provides that the court, in setting the fine within the guideline fine range, should consider any collateral consequences of conviction, including civil obligations arising from the organizations' conduct. As a general rule, collateral consequences that merely make victims whole provide no basis for reducing the fine within the guideline range. If criminal and civil sanctions are unlikely to make victims whole, this may provide a basis for a higher fine within the guideline fine range. If punitive collateral sanctions have been or will be imposed on the organization, this may provide a basis for a lower fine within the guideline fine range.

3. Subsection (a)(4) provides that the court, in setting the fine within the guideline fine range, should consider any nonpecuniary loss caused or threatened by the offense. To the extent that nonpecuniary loss caused or threatened (e.g., loss of or threat to human life; psychological injury; threat to national security) by the offense is not adequately considered in setting the guideline fine range, this factor provides a basis for a higher fine within the range. This factor is more likely to be applicable where the guideline fine range is determined by pecuniary loss or gain, rather than by offense level, because the Chapter Two offense levels frequently take actual or threatened nonpecuniary loss into account.

4. Subsection (a) (6) provides that the court, in setting the fine within the guideline fine range, should consider any prior criminal record of an individual within high-level personnel of the organization or a unit of the organization. Since an individual within high-level personnel either exercises substantial control over the organization or a unit of the organization or has a substantial role in the making of policy within the organization or a unit of the organization, any prior criminal misconduct of such an individual may be relevant to the determination of the appropriate fine for the organization.

5. Subsection (a)(7) provides that the court, in setting the fine within the guideline fine range, should consider any prior civil or criminal misconduct by the organization other than that counted under § 8C2.5(c). The civil and criminal misconduct counted under § 8C2.5(c) increases the guideline fine range. Civil or criminal misconduct other than that counted under § 8C2.5(c) may provide a basis for a higher fine within the range. In a case involving a pattern of illegality, an upward departure may be warranted.

6. Subsection (a) (8) provides that the court, in setting the fine within the guideline fine range, should consider any culpability score higher than ten or lower than zero. As the culpability score increases above ten, this may provide a basis for a higher fine within the range. Similarly, as the culpability score decreases below zero, this may provide a basis for a lower fine within the range.

7. Under subsection (b), the court, in determining the fine within the range, may consider any factor that it considered in determining the range. This allows for courts to differentiate between cases that have the same offense level but differ in seriousness (e.g., two fraud cases at offense level 12, one resulting in a loss of $21,000, the other $40,000). Similarly, this allows for courts to differentiate between two cases that have the same aggravating factors, but in which those factors vary in their intensity (e.g., two cases with upward adjustments to the culpability score under § 8C2.5(c)(2) (prior criminal adjudications within 5 years of the commencement of the instant offense, one involving a single conviction, the other involving two or more convictions).

Background: Subsection (a) includes factors that the court is required to consider under 18 U.S.C. 3553(a) and 3572(a) as well as additional factors that the Commission has determined may be relevant in a particular case. A number of factors required for consideration under 18 U.S.C. 3572(a) (e.g., pecuniary loss, the size of the organization) are used under the fine guidelines in this subpart to determine the fine range, and therefore are not specifically set out again in subsection (a) of this guideline. In unusual cases, factors listed in this section may provide a basis for departure.

§ 8C2.9. Disgorgement

The court shall add to the fine determined under § 8C2.8 (Determining the Fine Within the Range) any gain to the organization from the offense that has not and will not be paid as restitution or by way of other remedial measures.

25

Commentary

Application Note

1. This section is designed to ensure that the amount of any gain that has not and will not be taken from the organization for remedial purposes will be added to the fine. This section typically will apply in cases in which the organization has received gain from an offense but restitution or remedial efforts will not be required because the offense did not result in harm to identifiable victims, e.g., money laundering, obscenity, and regulatory reporting offenses. Money spent or to be spent to remedy the adverse effects of the offense, e.g., the cost to retrofit defective products, should be considered as disgorged gain. If the cost of remedial efforts made or to be made by the organization equals or exceeds the gain from the offense, this section will not apply.

§ 8C2.10. Determining the Fine for Other Counts

For any count or counts not covered under § 8C2.1 (Applicability of Fine Guidelines), the court should determine an appropriate fine by applying the provisions of 18 U.S.C. 3553 and 3572. The court should determine the appropriate fine amount, if any, to be imposed in addition to any fine determined under § 8C2.8 (Determining the Fine Within the Range) and § 8C2.9 (Disgorgement).

Commentary

Background: The Commission has not promulgated guidelines governing the setting of fines for counts not covered by § 8C2.1 (Applicability of Fine Guidelines). For such counts, the court should determine the appropriate fine based on the general statutory provisions governing sentencing. In cases that have a count or counts not covered by the guidelines in addition to a count or counts covered by the guidelines, the court shall apply the fine guidelines for the count(s) covered by the guidelines, and add any additional amount to the fine, as appropriate, for the count(s) not covered by the guidelines.

3. Implementing the Sentence of a Fine

§ 8C3.1. Imposing a Fine

(a) Except to the extent restricted by the maximum fine authorized by statute or any minimum fine required by statute, the fine or fine range shall be that determined under § 8C1.1 (Determining the Fine — Criminal Purpose Organizations); § 8C2.7 (Guideline Fine Range — Organizations) and § 8C2.9 (Disgorgement); or § 8C2.10 (Determining the Fine for Other Counts), as appropriate.

26

(b) Where the minimum guideline fine is greater than the maximum fine authorized by statute, the maximum fine authorized by statute shall be the guideline fine.

(c) Where the maximum guideline fine is less than a minimum fine required by statute, the minimum fine required by statute shall be the guideline fine.

Commentary

Background: This section sets forth the interaction of the fines or fine ranges determined under this chapter with the maximum fine authorized by statute and any minimum fine required by statute for the count or counts of conviction. The general statutory provisions governing a sentence of a fine are set forth in 18 U.S.C. 3571(c).

When the organization is convicted of multiple counts, the maximum fine authorized by statute may increase. For example, in the case of an organization convicted of three felony counts related to a $200,000 fraud, the maximum fine authorized by statute will be $500,000 on each count, for an aggregate maximum authorized fine of $1,500,000.

§ 8C3.2. Payment of the Fine — Organizations

(a) If the defendant operated primarily for a criminal purpose or primarily by criminal means, immediate payment of the fine shall be required.

(b) In any other case, immediate payment of the fine shall be required unless the court finds that the organization is financially unable to make immediate payment or that such payment would pose an undue burden on the organization. If the court permits other than immediate payment, it shall require full payment at the earliest possible date, either by requiring payment on a date certain or by establishing an installment schedule.

Commentary

Application Note

1. When the court permits other than immediate payment, the period provided for payment shall in no event exceed five years. 18 U.S.C. 3572(d).

§ 8C3.3. Reduction of Fine Based on Inability to Pay

(a) The court shall reduce the fine below that otherwise required by § 8C1.I (Determining the Fine — Criminal Purpose Organizations), or § 8C2.7 (Guideline Fine

Range — Organizations) and § 8C2.9 (Disgorgement), to the extent that imposition of such fine would impair its ability to make restitution to victims.

(b) The court may impose a fine below that otherwise required by § 8C2.7 (Guideline Fine Range — Organizations) and § 8C2.9 (Disgorgement) if the court finds that the organization is not able and, even with the use of a reasonable installment schedule, is not likely to become able to pay the minimum fine required by § 8C2.7 (Guideline Fine Range — Organizations) and § 8C2.9 (Disgorgement).

Provided, that the reduction under this subsection shall not be more than necessary to avoid substantially jeopardizing the continued viability of the organization.

Commentary

Application Note

1. For purposes of this section, an organization is not able to pay the minimum fine if even with an installment schedule under § 8C3.2 (Payment of the Fine — Organizations), the payment of that fine would substantially jeopardize the continued existence of the organization.

Background: Subsection (a) carries out the requirement in 18 U.S.C. 3572(b) that the court impose a fine or other monetary penalty only to the extent that such fine or penalty will not impair the ability of the organization to make restitution for the offense; however, this section does not authorize a criminal purpose organization to remain in business in order to pay restitution.

§ 8C3.4. Fines Paid by Owners of Closely-Held Organizations

The court may offset the fine imposed upon a closely-held organization when one or more individuals, each of whom owns at least a 5 percent interest in the organization, has been fined in a federal criminal proceeding for the same offense conduct for which the organization is being sentenced. The amount of such offset shall not exceed the amount resulting from multiplying the total fines imposed on those individuals by those individuals' total percentage interest in the organization.

Commentary

Application Notes

1. For purposes of this section, an organization is closely held, regardless of its size, when relatively few individuals own it. In order for an organization to be closely held, ownership and management need not completely overlap.

2. This section does not apply to a fine imposed upon an individual that arises out of offense conduct different from that for which the organization is being sentenced.

Background: For practical purposes, most closely-held organizations are the alter egos of their owner-managers. In the case of criminal conduct by a closely-held corporation, the organization and the culpable individual(s) both may be convicted. As a general rule in such cases, appropriate punishment may be achieved by offsetting the fine imposed upon the organization by an amount that reflects the percentage ownership interest of the sentenced individuals and the magnitude of the fines imposed upon those individuals. For example, an organization is owned by five individuals, each of whom has a twenty percent interest; three of the individuals are convicted; and the combined fines imposed on those three equals $100,000. In this example, the fine imposed upon the organization may be offset by up to 60 percent of their combined fine amounts, i.e., by $60,000.

4. Departures From the Guideline Fine Range

Introductory Commentary

The statutory provisions governing departures are set forth in 18 U.S.C. 3553(b). Departure may be warranted if the court finds 'that there exists an aggravating or mitigating circumstance of a kind, or to a degree, not adequately taken into consideration by the Sentencing Commission in formulating the guidelines that should result in a sentence different from that described.' This subpart sets forth certain factors that, in connection with certain offenses, may not have been adequately taken into consideration by the guidelines. In deciding whether departure is warranted, the court should consider the extent to which that factor is adequately taken into consideration by the guidelines and the relative importance or substantiality of that factor in the particular case.

To the extent that any policy statement from chapter Five, part K (Departures) is relevant to the organization, a departure from the applicable guideline fine range may be warranted. Some factors listed in chapter Five, part K that are particularly applicable to organizations are listed in this subpart. Other factors listed in chapter Five, part K may be applicable in particular cases. While this subpart lists factors that the Commission believes may constitute grounds for departure, the list is not exhaustive.

§ 8C4.1. Substantial Assistance to Authorities — Organizations (Policy Statement)

(a) Upon motion of the government stating that the defendant has provided substantial assistance in the investigation or prosecution of another organization that has committed an offense, or in the investigation or prosecution of an individual not directly affiliated with the defendant who has committed an offense, the court may depart from the guidelines.

(b) The appropriate reduction shall be determined by the court for reasons stated on the record that may include, but are not limited to, consideration of the following:

(1) The court's evaluation of the significance and usefulness of the organization's assistance, taking into consideration the government's evaluation of the assistance rendered;

(2) The nature and extent of the organization's assistance; and

(3) The timeliness of the organization's assistance.

Commentary

Application Note

1. Departure under this section is intended for cases in which substantial assistance is provided in the investigation or prosecution of crimes committed by individuals not directly affiliated with the organization or by other organizations. It is not intended for assistance in the investigation or prosecution of the agents of the organization responsible for the offense for which the organization is being sentenced.

§ 8C4.2. Risk of Death or Bodily Injury (Policy Statement)

If the offense resulted in death or bodily injury, or involved a foreseeable risk of death or bodily injury, an upward departure may be warranted. The extent of any such departure should depend, among other factors, on the nature of the harm and the extent to which the harm was intended or knowingly risked, and the extent to which such harm or risk is taken into account within the applicable guideline fine range.

§ 8C4.3. Threat to National Security (Policy Statement)

If the offense constituted a threat to national security, an upward departure may be warranted.

§ 8C4.4. Threat to the Environment (Policy Statement)

If the offense presented a threat to the environment, an upward departure may be warranted.

§ 8C4.5. Threat to a Market (Policy Statement)

If the offense presented a risk to the integrity or continued existence of a market, an upward departure may be warranted. This section is applicable to both private markets (e.g., a financial market, a commodities market, or a market for consumer goods) and public markets (e.g., government contracting).

§ 8C4.6. Official Corruption (Policy Statement)

If the organization, in connection with the offense, bribed or unlawfully gave a gratuity to a public official, or attempted or conspired to bribe or unlawfully give a gratuity to a public official, an upward departure may be warranted.

§ 8C4.7. Public Entity (Policy Statement)

If the organization is a public entity, a downward departure may be warranted.

§ 8C4.8. Members or Beneficiaries of the Organization as Victims (Policy Statement)

If the members or beneficiaries, other than shareholders, of the organization are direct victims of the offense, a downward departure may be warranted. If the members or beneficiaries of an organization are direct victims of the offense, imposing a fine upon the organization may increase the burden upon the victims of the offense without achieving a deterrent effect. In such cases, a fine may not be appropriate. For example, departure may be appropriate if a labor union is convicted of embezzlement of pension funds.

§ 8C4.9. Remedial Costs that Greatly Exceed Gain (Policy Statement)

If the organization has paid or has agreed to pay remedial costs arising from the offense that greatly exceed the gain that the organization received from the offense, a downward departure may be warranted. In such a case, a substantial fine may not be necessary in order to achieve adequate punishment and deterrence. In deciding whether departure is appropriate, the court should consider the level and extent of substantial authority personnel involvement in the offense and the degree to which the loss exceeds the gain. If an individual within high-level personnel was involved in the offense, a departure would not be appropriate under this section. The lower the level and the more limited the extent of substantial authority personnel involvement in the offense, and the greater the degree to which remedial costs exceeded or will exceed gain, the less will be the need for a substantial fine to achieve adequate punishment and deterrence.

§ 8C4.10. Mandatory Programs to Prevent and Detect Violations of Law (Policy Statement)

If the organization's culpability score is reduced under § 8C2.5(f) (Effective Program to Prevent and Detect Violations of Law) and the organization had implemented its program in response to a court order or administrative order specifically directed at the organization, an upward departure may be warranted to offset, in part or in whole, such reduction.

§ 8C4.11. Exceptional Organizational Culpability (Policy Statement)

If the organization's culpability score is greater than 10, an upward departure may be appropriate.

If no individual within substantial authority personnel participated in, condoned, or was willfully ignorant of the offense; the organization at the time of the offense bad an effective program to prevent and detect violations of law; and the base fine is determined under §§ 8C2.4(a)(1), 8C2.4(a)(3), or a special instruction for fines in Chapter Two (Offense Conduct), a downward departure may be warranted. In a case meeting these criteria, the court may find that the organization had exceptionally low culpability and therefore a fine based on loss, offense level, or a special Chapter Two instruction results in a guideline fine range higher than necessary to achieve the purposes of sentencing. Nevertheless, such fine should not be lower than if determined under § 8C2.4(a)(2).

Part D — Organizational Probation

Introductory Commentary

Section 8D1.1 sets forth the circumstances under which a sentence to a term of probation is required. Sections 8D1.2 through 8D1.5 address the length of the probation term, conditions of probation, and violations of probation conditions.

32

§ 8D1.1. Imposition of Probation — Organizations

(a) The court shall order a term of probation:

(1) If such sentence is necessary to secure payment of restitution (§ 8B1.1), enforce a remedial order (§ 8B1.2), or ensure completion of community service (§ 8B1.3);

(2) If the organization is sentenced to pay a monetary penalty (e.g., restitution, fine, or special assessment), the penalty is not paid in full at the time of sentencing, and restrictions are necessary to safeguard the organization's ability to make payments;

(3) If at the time of sentencing, an organization having 50 or more employees does not have an effective program to prevent and detect violations of law;

(4) If the organization within five years prior to sentencing engaged in similar misconduct, as determined by a prior criminal adjudication, and any part of the misconduct underlying the instant offense occurred after that adjudication;

(5) If an individual within high-level personnel of the organization or the unit of the organization within which the instant offense was committed participated in the misconduct underlying the instant offense and that individual within five years prior to sentencing engaged in similar misconduct, as determined by a prior criminal adjudication, and any part of the misconduct underlying the instant offense occurred after that adjudication;

(6) If such sentence is necessary to ensure that changes are made within the organization to reduce the likelihood of future criminal conduct;

(7) If the sentence imposed upon the organization does not include a fine; or

(8) If necessary to accomplish one or more of the purposes of sentencing set forth in 18 U.S.C. 3553(a)(2).

Commentary

Background: Under 18 U.S.C. 3561(a), an organization may be sentenced to a term of probation. Under 18 U.S.C. 3551(c), imposition of a term of probation is required if the sentence imposed upon the organization does not include a fine.

§ 8D1.2. Term of Probation — Organizations

(a) When a sentence of probation is imposed —

(1) In the case of a felony, the term of probation shall be at least one year but not more than five years.

(2) In any other case, the term of probation shall be not more than five years.

Commentary

Application Note

1. Within the limits set by the guidelines, the term of probation should be sufficient, but not more than necessary, to accomplish the court's specific objectives in imposing the term of probation. The terms of probation set forth in this section are those provided in 18 U.S.C. 3561(b).

§ 8D1.3. Conditions of Probation — Organizations

(a) Pursuant to 18 U.S.C. 3563(a)(1), any sentence of probation shall include the condition that the organization shall not commit another federal, state, or local crime during the term of probation.

(b) Pursuant to 18 U.S.C. 3563(a)(2), if a sentence of probation is imposed for a felony, the court shall impose as a condition of probation at least one of the following: A fine, restitution, or community service, unless the court finds on the record that extraordinary circumstances exist that would make such condition plainly unreasonable, in which event the court shall impose one or more other conditions set forth in 18 U.S.C. 3563(b).

(c) The court may impose other conditions that (1) are reasonably related to the nature and circumstances of the offense or the history and characteristics of the organization; and (2) involve only such deprivations of liberty or property as are necessary to effect the purposes of sentencing.

§ 8D1.4. Recommended Conditions of Probation — Organizations (Policy Statement)

(a) The court may order the organization, at its expense and in the format and media specified by the court, to publicize the nature of the offense committed, the fact of conviction, the nature of the punishment imposed, and the steps that will be taken to prevent the recurrence of similar offenses.

(b) If probation is imposed under § 8D1.1(a)(2), the following conditions may be appropriate to the extent they appear necessary to safeguard the organization's ability to pay any deferred portion of an order of restitution, fine, or assessment:

(1) The organization shall make periodic submissions to the court or probation officer, at intervals specified by the court, reporting on the organization's financial condition and results of business operations, and accounting for the disposition of all funds received.

(2) The organization shall submit to: (A) A reasonable number of regular or unannounced examinations of its books and records at appropriate business premises by the probation officer or experts engaged by the court; and (B) interrogation of knowledgeable individuals within the organization. Compensation to and costs of any experts engaged by the court shall be paid by the organization.

(3) The organization shall be required to notify the court or probation officer immediately upon learning of (A) any material adverse change in its business or financial condition or prospects, or (B) the commencement of any bankruptcy proceeding, major civil litigation, criminal prosecution, or administrative proceeding against the organization, or any investigation or formal inquiry by governmental authorities regarding the organization.

(4) The organization shall be required to make periodic payments, as specified by the court, in the following priority: (1) Restitution; (2) fine; and (3) any other monetary sanction.

(c) If probation is ordered under § 8D1.1(a) (3), (4), (5), or (6), the following conditions may be appropriate:

(1) The organization shall develop and submit to the court a program to prevent and detect violations of law, including a schedule for implementation.

(2) Upon approval by the court of a program to prevent and detect violations of law, the organization shall notify its employees and shareholders of its criminal behavior and its program to prevent and detect violations of law. Such notice shall be in a form prescribed by the court.

(3) The organization shall make periodic reports to the court or probation officer, at intervals and in a form specified by the court, regarding the organization's progress in implementing the program to prevent and detect violations of law. Among other things, such reports shall disclose any criminal prosecution, civil litigation, or administrative

proceeding commenced against the organization, or any investigation or formal inquiry by governmental authorities of which the organization learned since its last report.

(4) In order to monitor whether the organization is following the program to prevent and detect violations of law, the organization shall submit to: (A) A reasonable number of regular or unannounced examinations of its books and records at appropriate business premises by the probation officer or experts engaged by the court; and (B) interrogation of knowledgeable individuals within the organization. Compensation to and costs of any experts engaged by the court shall be paid by the organization.

Commentary

Application Notes

1. In determining the conditions to be imposed when probation is ordered under § 8D1.1(a) (3) through (6), the court should consider the views of any governmental regulatory body that oversees conduct of the organization relating to the instant offense. To assess the efficacy of a program submitted by the organization, the court may employ appropriate experts who shall be afforded access to all material possessed by the organization that is necessary for a comprehensive assessment of the proposed program. The court should approve any program that appears reasonably calculated to prevent and detect violations of law, provided it is consistent with any applicable statutory or regulatory requirement.

2. Periodic reports submitted in accordance with subsection (c)(3) should be provided to any governmental regulatory body that oversees conduct of the organization relating to the instant offense.

§ 8D1.5. Violations of Conditions of Probation — Organizations (Policy Statement)

Upon a finding of a violation of a condition of probation, the court may extend the term of probation, impose more restrictive conditions of probation, or revoke probation and resentence the organization.

Commentary

Application Note

1. In the event of repeated, serious violations of conditions of probation, the appointment of a master or trustee may be appropriate to ensure compliance with court orders.

Part E — Special Assessments, Forfeitures, and Costs § 8E1.1. Special Assessments — Organizations

A special assessment must be imposed on an organization in the amount prescribed by statute.

Commentary

Background: Pursuant to 18 U.S.C. 3013(a), the court is required to impose assessments in the following amounts:

$50, if the organization is convicted of a Class B misdemeanor;
$125, if the organization is convicted of a Class A misdemeanor; and
$200, if the organization is convicted of a felony. 18 U.S.C. 3013.

The Act does not authorize the court to waive imposition of the assessment.

§ 8E1.2. Forfeiture — Organizations

Apply § 5E1.4 (Forfeiture).

§ 8E1.3. Assessment of Costs — Organizations

As provided in 28 U.S.C. 1918, the court may order the organization to pay the costs of prosecution. In addition, specific statutory provisions mandate assessment of costs.

Section 2B4.1 is amended by inserting the following additional subsection:

"(c) Special Instruction for Fines — Organizations.

In lieu of the pecuniary loss under subsection (a)(3) of § 8C2.4 (Base Fine), use the greatest of: (1) the value of the unlawful payment; (2) the value of the benefit received or to be received in return for the unlawful payment; or (3) the consequential damages resulting from the unlawful payment."

Section 2C1.1 is amended by inserting the following additional subsection:

"(d) Special Instruction for Fines — Organizations.

In lieu of the pecuniary loss under subsection (a)(3) of § 8C2.4 (Base Fine), use the greatest of: (I) the value of the unlawful payment; (2) the value of the benefit received or to be received in return for the unlawful payment; or (3) the consequential damag resulting from the unlawful payment."

Section 2C1.2 is amended by inserting the following additional subsection:

"(c) Special Instruction for Fines — Organizations.

In lieu of the pecuniary loss under subsection, (a) (3) of § 8C2.4 (Base Fine), u the value of the unlawful payment.

Section 2E5.1 is amended by inserting the following additional subsection:

"(c) Special Instruction for Fines — Organizations.

In lieu of the pecuniary loss under subsection (a) (3) of § 8C2.4 (Base Fine), use t greatest of: (1) the value of the unlawful payment; (2) if a bribe, the value of the bene received or to be received in return for the unlawful payment; or (3) if a bribe, t consequential damages resulting from the unlawful payment."

Section 2E5.6 is amended by inserting the following additional subsection:

"(c) Special Instruction for Fines — Organizations.

In lieu of the pecuniary loss under subsection (a)(3) of § 8C2.4 (Base Fine), use t greatest of: (1) the value of the unlawful payment; (2) if a bribe, the value of the bene received or to be received in return for the unlawful payment; or (3) if a bribe, t consequential damages resulting from the unlawful payment."

The Commentary to section 2F1.1 captioned "Application Notes" is amended Application Note 7 by inserting the following penultimate paragraph:

"For offenses involving diversion of government program payments, loss is the valu of the monetary benefits diverted from intended recipients or uses.

Section 2R1.1 is amended by inserting the following additional subsection:

(d) Special Instructions for Fines — Organizations.

(1) In lieu of the pecuniary loss under subsection (a) (3) of § 8C2.4 (Bas Fine), use 20 percent of the volume of affected commerce.

(2) When applying § 8C2.6 (Minimum and Maximum Multipliers), neithe the minimum nor maximum multiplier shall be less than 0.75.

(3) In a bid-rigging case in which the organization submitted one or more complementary bids, use as the organization's volume of commerce the greater of (A) the volume of commerce done by the organization in the goods or services that were affected by the violation, or (B) the largest contract on which the organization submitted a complementary bid in connection with the bid-rigging conspiracy."

The Commentary to § 2R1.1 captioned "Application Notes" is amended by deleting Application Note 3 and inserting in lieu thereof:

"3. The fine for an organization is determined by applying Chapter Eight (Sentencing of Organizations). In selecting a fine for an organization within the guideline fine range, the court should consider both the gain to the organization from the offense and the loss caused by the organization. It is estimated that the average gain from price-fixing is 10 percent of the selling price. The loss from price-fixing exceeds the gain because, inter alia, injury is inflicted upon consumers who are unable or for other reasons do not buy the product at the higher prices. Because the loss from price-fixing exceeds the gain, subsection (d)(1) provides that 20 percent of the volume of affected commerce is to be used in lieu of the pecuniary loss under § 8C2.4(a)(3). The purpose for specifying a percent of the volume of commerce is to avoid the time and expense that would be required for the court to determine the actual gain or loss. In cases in which the actual monopoly overcharge appears to be either substantially more or substantially less than 10 percent, this factor should be considered in setting the fine within the guideline fine range."

The Commentary to § 2R.1 is amended by deleting the final paragraph of Background and inserting in lieu thereof:

"Substantial fines are an essential part of the sentence. For an individual, the guideline fine range is from one to five percent of the volume of commerce, but not less than $20,000. For an organization, the guideline fine range is determined under Chapter Eight (Sentencing of Organizations), but pursuant to subsection (d)(2), the minimum multiplier is 0.75. This multiplier allows a minimum fine of 15 percent of the volume of commerce for the least serious case. The minimum multiplier of 0.75 was selected to provide an effective deterrent to antitrust offenses. At the same time, this minimum multiplier maintains incentives for desired organizational behavior. Because the Department of justice has a well-established amnesty program for organizations that self-report antitrust offenses, no lower minimum multiplier is needed as an incentive for self-reporting. A minimum multiplier of 0.75 ensures that fines imposed in antitrust cases will exceed the average monopoly overcharge.

The Commission believes that most antitrust defendants have the resources and earning capacity to pay the fines called for by this guideline, at least over time on an installment basis. The statutory maximum fine is $350,000 for individuals and $1,000,000 for organizations, but is increased when there are convictions on multiple counts."

Section 251.1 is amended by inserting the following additional subsection:

39

"(c) Special Instructions for Fines — Organizations.

In lieu of the applicable amount from the table in subsection (d) of § 8C2.4 (Base Fine), use:

(1) The greater of $250,000 or 100 percent of the value of the funds if subsections (a)(1) and (b)(1) are used to determine the offense level; or

(2) The greater of $200,000 or 70 percent of the value of the funds if subsections (a)(2) and (b)(1) are used to determine the offense level; or

(3) The greater of $200,000 or 70 percent of the value of the funds if subsection (a)(1) but not (b)(1) is used to determine the offense level; or

(4) The greater of $150,000 or 50 percent of the value of the funds if subsection (a)(2) but not (b)(1) is used to determine the offense level.

Section 2S1.2 is amended by inserting the following additional subsection:

"(c) Special Instructions for Fines — Organizations.

In lieu of the applicable amount from the table in subsection (d) of § 8C2.4 (Base Fine), use:

(1) The greater of $175,000 or 60 percent of the value of the funds if subsection (b)(1)(A) is used to determine the offense level; or

(2) The greater of $150,000 or 50 percent of the value of the funds if subsection (b)(1)(B) is used to determine the offense level."

Section 2S1.3 is amended by inserting the following additional subsection:

"(c) Special Instructions for Fines — Organizations.

In lieu of the applicable amount from the table in subsection (d) of § 8C2.4 (Base Fine), use:

(1) The greater of $125,000 or 30 percent of the value of the funds if subsections (a)(1) and (b)(1) are used to determine the offense level; or

(2) The greater of $50,000 or 20 percent of the value of the funds if subsection (a)(1) but not (b)(1) is used to determine the offense level."

Section 2S1.4 is amended by inserting the following additional subsection:

"(c) Special Instructions for Fines — Organizations.

In lieu of the applicable amount from the table in subsection (d) of § 8C2.4 (Base Fine), use:

(1) The greater of $50,000 or 20 percent of the value of the funds if subsection (b)(I) or (b)(2) is used to determine the offense level; or

(2) The greater of $15,000 or 10 percent of the value of the funds, otherwise."

Reason for the Amendment: Pursuant to its authority and in accord with its responsibilities under 28 U.S.C. 994(a), the Commission has promulgated guidelines and policy statements for the sentencing of organizational defendants. The Commentary contained within Chapter Eight, particularly the Introductory and Background Commentary, provides a basic statement of the reasons for the Commission's recommendations. [FR Doc. 91-11258 Filed 5-15-91; 8:45 A.M.]